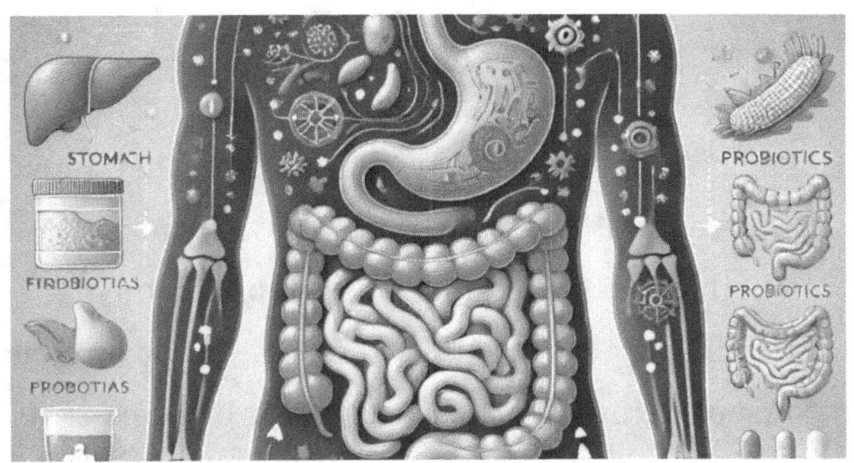

Gut Health Revolution

Transform Your Life with a Balanced Microbiome

Verna B. Hagen

COPYRIGHT PAGE

DISCLAIMER PAGE

This book is intended for educational purposes only and should not be considered a replacement for professional medical advice, diagnosis, or treatment. Before making any changes to your diet, exercise routine, or treatment plan, always consult with a healthcare professional.

The author and publisher are not liable for any negative outcomes or consequences arising from the use of the information in this book. Results may differ from person to person, and the content should not be used as a substitute for professional medical consultation.

Table of Contents

INTRODUCTION

Gut health is a revolution in our understanding of the inner workings of our bodies, not merely a trendy term. Often called the body's "second brain," the stomach affects every facet of our health. The digestive system, immunity, mental clarity, weight control, and even our mood is all influenced by the gut.

However, many people are not aware of how much their gut affects their general health, despite its significance.

The gut microbiome, which is made up of billions of bacteria, viruses, fungus, and other microorganisms, lives in your gut. Your physical and emotional wellbeing are greatly impacted by this intricate network. Your body's ability to digest food, absorb nutrients, and fend off dangerous diseases is influenced by the condition of your gut microbiome. It also has an unexpected relationship with your brain, affecting your mental health, stress levels, and mood.

A variety of health problems, from digestive issues like bloating and IBS to more serious conditions like autoimmune diseases, chronic inflammation, and mental health disorders like anxiety and depression, can be caused by an imbalance in the gut microbiome, which is regrettably a result of modern lifestyles, poor diets, stress, and environmental factors.

The purpose of this book is to assist you in navigating this revolution in gut health. Understanding the science behind your gut and how it affects your health is the first step towards regaining control, regardless of whether you've battled with mood swings, chronic digestive problems, inexplicable exhaustion, or brain fog.

You will learn how to restore equilibrium and enhance not only your digestion but also your general health by concentrating on the stomach, which is the primary culprit. This book provides useful advice, scientific insights, and doable tactics to improve, maintain, and heal your gut. To improve the way you feel, think, and live, you need to make long-lasting adjustments to your food, lifestyle, and thinking. It's not just about knowing about your gut.

How to Utilize This Manual

This article is designed to give you practical advice based on validated research so you may gradually improve the health of your gut. From the gut microbiota to the gut-brain connection, each chapter delves into a different facet of gut health and provides easy-to-implement solutions that you may use on a daily basis.

- To establish a solid foundation for gut health, start at the beginning.
- Take your time, experimenting with dietary, lifestyle, and habit modifications.
- Monitor your development and make any corrections. It's about development and consistency, not perfection.

This Guide's Objective

This guide's goal is straightforward: to provide you with the information and resources you need to take charge of your gut health. You can make decisions that are good for your body and mind if you know how your stomach works and how it relates to your general health.

This book offers helpful, doable actions that can help you recover, feel better, and lead a more active life in addition to knowledge. This book will assist you in making long-lasting changes, whether your goal is to enhance your mood, increase your energy, or address digestive problems.

How You Will Benefit from This Guide

You will be able to:

Recognize how important the gut microbiota is for immunity, digestion, and mental health by using the advice and techniques in this guide.

Discover how to include foods that are good for your gut, such as probiotics and prebiotics, in your diet.

Learn about the strong link between gut health and mood management, brain function, and weight loss.

To enhance gut health, employ doable tactics like stress reduction and intermittent fasting.

Acquire the resources necessary to design a customized gut health plan that meets your requirements and lifestyle.

In addition to giving, you a greater understanding of your body, this guide will give you a clear road map for long-term health improvement.

A Patient's Journey: An Account of Change

For years, I battled stomach problems, persistent exhaustion, and erratic mood swings. I felt trapped in a loop of ineffective therapies and medications that never appeared to address the underlying cause of my issues, even after seeing multiple doctors.

Next, I discovered Dr. Verna B. Hagen. I came to the conclusion that my digestive problems were probably related to an imbalance in my gut microbiota after reading her observations and learning about the significant influence the gut has on general health. The first step to recovery was coming to this realization.

Under Dr. Hagen's direction, I started making little but significant adjustments. I started intermittent fasting, concentrated on lowering stress, and changed my diet to incorporate more probiotics and prebiotics. My health significantly improved as a result of these minor adjustments. My energy levels rose, my mood stabilized, and my digestion became more regular.

In addition to offering me short-term respite, Dr. Hagen's method helped me identify the underlying cause of my issues and equipped me with the means to create long-lasting improvements. I felt like I had real control over my health for the first time in years.

Part 1: Unlocking the Secrets of the Gut

CHAPTER 1

The Hidden World of Gut Microbiome

An invisible world—an ecosystem—resides in your gut and is crucial to your overall health. The gut is home to a vibrant colony of billions of microscopic bacteria, despite the fact that we frequently concentrate on the organs that are visible, such as the heart, lungs, and brain.

The gut microbiome is made up of these microorganisms, which include bacteria, viruses, fungi, and even some parasites. They may or may not coexist peacefully inside your digestive tract.

Like an internal jungle, the gut microbiome is teeming with many living forms, each of which has a distinct function. Your gut microbiome is crucial for preserving balance in your body, much like the ecosystem of a rainforest is for preserving equilibrium in the natural world. It's amazing to consider that there are almost ten times as many of these minuscule organisms as human cells. And more intriguing still? They affect almost every bodily system, including your weight, immunity, digestion, and mental wellness.

What is the gut microbiome exactly?

The trillions of bacteria that live in your gastrointestinal tract, mostly in the large intestine, are collectively referred to as your gut microbiome. This encompasses a wide range of microorganisms, including viruses, fungi, archaea, and bacteria, both beneficial and harmful. The microbiome is sometimes referred to as the "forgotten organ" due to its significant impact on physiological processes that humans frequently ignore.

The microbiome of every individual is distinct and influenced by a number of variables, such as environment, age, genetics, and food. At different stages of life, the microbiome balance in your gut might differ significantly from that of another person and even from your own. The intriguing thing about personalized health is that no two microbiomes are alike.

For thousands of years, the microbiome has changed in tandem with humans. However, this fragile ecosystem has been upset in the contemporary era by stress, food, antibiotic usage, and changes in lifestyle. Although the study of the microbiome's effects on health is still in its infancy, it is expanding quickly. Let's examine these invisible organisms' effects on your body in more detail.

The Impact of Your Gut Microbiota on Your Health

1. Digestion: The Function of the Gut as the Body's Processing Facility

Your mouth performs the initial stage of digestion when you eat, but your stomach and intestines do the bulk of the work. In this process, the gut microbiota plays a significant role. Complex carbs, fibers, and even certain proteins that your body is unable to digest on its own are broken down with its assistance.

For instance, people lack the enzymes necessary to break down fiber, despite the fact that it is necessary for healthy digestion and regular bowel movements. Let's talk about the microbiota. Fiber can be fermented by specific gut bacteria to produce short-chain fatty acids such as propionate, acetate, and butyrate. These short-chain fatty acids contain anti-inflammatory properties, maintain the integrity of the gut lining, and give your gut cells energy.

Your digestion might not be as effective if your gut microbiota is out of balance. Bloating, constipation, diarrhea, and illnesses like irritable bowel syndrome (IBS) might result from this.

2. Immunity: The Body's Immune Fortress

The gut microbiota is frequently referred to as the "second brain" because of its impact on your brain and immune system. In actuality, the stomach contains over 70% of your immune system. Your body's immunological responses are developed and regulated in large part by the microorganisms in your digestive system.

These microorganisms teach your immune system to discriminate between benign substances (like food or beneficial bacteria) and dangerous intruders (like bacteria or viruses). The immune system's capacity to fight off infections and stop inflammatory reactions is strengthened by a balanced, healthy microbiome.

However, an unbalanced microbiome, commonly referred to as dysbiosis, can lead to persistent inflammation, which weakens your immune system and increases your risk of attacking your own tissues. This is the characteristic of autoimmune diseases like Crohn's disease and rheumatoid arthritis.

Furthermore, the growth of T-cells and the synthesis of antibodies—both crucial for immunological regulation—are influenced by the gut microbiota. In addition to reducing inflammation and preventing infections, a healthy microbiome may potentially affect how well vaccines work.

3. Mental Health: The Link Between the Gut and the Brain

The connection between the gut and the brain is among the most fascinating findings of the last few years. The phrase "gut-brain axis" was created by researchers to refer to the ongoing exchange of information between the central nervous system and the gut. It turns out that your attitude, emotions, and cognitive abilities can all be directly impacted by the bacteria that reside in your gut. The brain requires a number of compounds produced by the gut microbiota, including dopamine, gamma-aminobutyric acid (GABA), which helps control anxiety, and serotonin, the "feel-good" neurotransmitter. In actuality, the gut produces almost 90% of the serotonin in the body.

Therefore, an imbalance in your microbiome can alter the chemistry of your brain, which may result in diseases like anxiety, sadness, or even neurodevelopmental disorders like autism. The gut microbiota also plays a role in controlling the stress response. A healthy gut microbiome can contribute to better mental and emotional well-being by mitigating the negative effects of stress.

4. Weight Control: The Function of Your Gut in Metabolism

The fact that your gut microorganisms have a significant impact on how your body processes food and may even affect your weight may surprise you. The gut microbiota aids in nutrition absorption, food digestion, and metabolism regulation.

Certain gut bacterial species can affect how your body stores fat and are more adept at obtaining energy from meals than others. adults with an unbalanced microbiome may be more likely to be obese because of the excess of specific microorganisms that take more calories from food, according to a study done on obese adults. On the other hand, a healthy microbiome can lower the risk of weight gain and metabolic disorders like type 2 diabetes by regulating metabolism.

Your body's reaction to certain foods is also influenced by your microbiome. Whole grains, fiber-rich foods, and healthy fats are better absorbed by a gut microbiota that is in balance, which can help people lose weight and avoid obesity. Dysbiosis and weight gain can result from poor diets, particularly those heavy in processed foods and sugar.

5. Inflammation and the Prevention of Disease

The condition of your digestive system The microbiome is crucial in controlling inflammation in the body as a whole. Chronic low-grade inflammation, which is a risk factor for numerous illnesses, such as diabetes, cancer, and heart disease, can result from an imbalance in the bacteria community in your gut.

By generating anti-inflammatory substances like short-chain fatty acids that support the integrity of the gut lining, a healthy gut microbiota helps avoid excessive inflammation. This helps avoid the disease known as "leaky gut," in which the lining of the stomach becomes permeable, enabling toxic compounds to enter the bloodstream and causing inflammation.

According to studies, those who have an unbalanced microbiome are more prone to autoimmune disorders, allergies, and inflammatory bowel disease (IBD). One way to lower the risk of these autoimmune and inflammatory diseases is to support a healthy gut microbiota.

Your Health and Your Microbiome
A strong and intricate system, the gut microbiota affects almost every facet of your health. These microscopic creatures affect many aspects of your daily life, including digestion, immune system performance, mental health, and even weight regulation. The more we understand about the

microbiome, the more obvious it is that overall health depends on having a balanced, healthy gut. For this reason, maintaining the health of your gut should be your first priority. You can cultivate and nourish your microbiome by making little adjustments to your diet, lifestyle, and behaviors. This will improve your digestion, boost your immunity, elevate your mood, and sharpen your mind.

Although the gut microbiome's science is still developing, one thing is clear: the secret to a happier, healthier existence lies in this hidden world inside of us.

CHAPTER 2

Your Gut: The Body's Command Center

The immune system is probably the first thing that comes to mind when you think of your body's defenses. And while most people think of the spleen or lymph nodes when they think of immune systems, a big part of your immune system is actually in your gut. That's right, your gut does more than just digest food.

It also protects your body from external threats. People have even called the gut the "second brain" of the body because it has such a big impact on so many processes, including the immune system. A powerful way to understand how to improve your general health is to learn about the link between your gut and your immune system. The link comes from gut-associated lymphoid tissue (GALT), which is a big part of your immune system and lives in the lining of your digestive track.

Today, we're going to talk about how important your gut is for your immune system and how it helps keep you healthy and free of diseases, infections, and even long-term conditions like autoimmune disorders.

Your gut is where your immune system starts. Approximately 70-80% of your immune cells are found in your gastrointestinal system. These cells are constantly on the lookout, scanning the food you eat, the bacteria that reside in your gut, and any possible harmful pathogens that could threaten your health. If your gut microbiome is in balance, your immune system can successfully protect you from external threats like viruses, bacteria, and even toxins. However, if the balance is disrupted (a situation called dysbiosis), it can lead to a weakened immune reaction, making you more susceptible to illness.

But why does your gut contain such a big proportion of your immune system? It all comes down to the role your gut plays as your body's first line of defense. Everything you consume—food, water, and air—enters through the gut, so it makes sense that your immune system would be focused here. When your body recognizes harmful invaders in your digestive system, like pathogens or toxins, your gut activates immune responses to neutralize or remove them.

Gut-Immune Connection: The Role of the Microbiome

The microbiome plays an important part in maintaining this immune function. It's not just about bacteria that help digest food; it's about the ongoing communication between the microbes and your immune system. A well-balanced microbiome can help "train" your immune system to distinguish between dangerous pathogens and harmless substances (like food or friendly bacteria), so your body doesn't overreact or cause unnecessary inflammation.

Healthy gut flora—the group of beneficial microbes in your gut—produces compounds that help regulate immune reactions. They support the gut lining, making it more resistant to pathogens, and help create a balanced inflammatory reaction. When the microbiome is imbalanced, however, this process goes awry, possibly leading to chronic inflammation, an overactive immune response, or even autoimmune diseases.

The Gut as the Body's "Alarm System"

Your gut works like an alarm system that signals your immune system when something is wrong. When pathogens or harmful substances enter your gut, they trigger your immune system to release cytokines—small signaling molecules that help coordinate the immune reaction. In this way, your gut can warn the rest of the body to danger, whether that's a pathogen, toxin, or even a foreign food protein that the immune system mistakenly attacks.

But what happens when the alarm system is tripped too often? The constant activation of your immune reaction can result in chronic inflammation, a condition that has been linked to numerous diseases, including heart disease, diabetes, arthritis, and even cancer. This is why keeping a healthy gut microbiome is so critical: when it is balanced, your immune system can operate effectively without triggering unnecessary inflammation.

Gut Health and Autoimmune Diseases

One of the most fascinating (and concerning) parts of the gut's immune function is its role in autoimmune diseases. Autoimmune diseases occur when the immune system mistakenly attacks the body's own cells. In conditions like rheumatoid arthritis, lupus, and multiple sclerosis, the immune system fails to recognize "self" from "non-self" and starts attacking healthy tissue.

Recent study has shown that an imbalanced gut microbiome can play a key role in the development of autoimmune diseases. The gut microbiota is involved in teaching the immune system to distinguish between harmless substances and threats.

When this education process is disrupted, the immune system may begin fighting the body's own cells, leading to autoimmune reactions. In fact, conditions such as inflammatory bowel disease (IBD) and celiac disease have been highly linked to gut health imbalances.

Some studies even suggest that dysbiosis, an imbalance of gut bacteria, could cause or exacerbate conditions like rheumatoid arthritis or type 1 diabetes, where the immune system attacks its own joints or pancreas. The good news? By restoring balance to the gut microbiome, these immune responses can often be modulated, lowering the severity of symptoms or possibly even reversing the progression of some autoimmune diseases.

How to Keep Your Gut Immune System Healthy

Maintaining a healthy gut and supporting your immune system doesn't have to be difficult. In fact, it starts with a few simple lifestyle changes that can greatly improve the health of both your gut and your immune system.

1. Eat a Diverse, Plant-Rich Diet

A diverse diet rich in whole foods—especially fruits, vegetables, whole grains, legumes, and fermented foods—helps promote a diverse gut microbiome, which is important for a balanced immune system. The different fibers and polyphenols found in plant-based foods fuel beneficial gut bacteria, which in turn helps control immune function.

Incorporating fermented foods like yogurt, kefir, sauerkraut, and kimchi can further boost gut health by introducing beneficial probiotics into the digestive system. These probiotics help balance the gut microbiome, avoiding the overgrowth of harmful bacteria that could impair immune function.

2. Avoid Overuse of Antibiotics

Antibiotics, while sometimes necessary for treating infections, can have a negative effect on the gut microbiome. They don't just kill harmful bacteria; they also wipe out beneficial bacteria that play a key role in immune health. When possible, it's important to limit the use of antibiotics and only take them when recommended by a healthcare provider.

3. Manage Stress

Chronic worry can wreak havoc on your gut and immune system. When you're worried, your body releases the hormone cortisol, which can disrupt the balance of gut bacteria and impair immune function. Stress also leads to inflammation, which can activate the immune system and add to chronic diseases. Practicing stress-reducing techniques like yoga, meditation, deep breathing, or simply taking time for yourself can help keep your gut and immune system in check.

4. Get Enough Sleep

Sleep is important for overall health, including gut health. Poor sleep has been linked to dysbiosis and weakened immune function. During sleep, your body is in repair mode, including healing your gut lining and restoring microbial balance. Aim for 7-9 hours of sleep each night to help your immune system to function optimally.

5. Exercise Regularly

Regular physical action has been shown to support gut health by promoting a diverse microbiome. Exercise helps lower inflammation and enhances the immune system's ability to respond to threats. Aim for at least 30 minutes of mild exercise most days of the week to keep your gut—and immune system—working at their best.

Your Gut, Your Immune System

The gut is undeniably important to your immune system and overall health. It serves as the first line of defense against harmful invaders, constantly monitoring and signaling the body's immune reaction. By maintaining a balanced gut microbiome through diet, lifestyle, and mindful habits, you can empower your immune system to work optimally, fight off infections, and avoid chronic diseases.

Taking care of your gut isn't just about avoiding stomach discomfort—it's about protecting and improving your body's natural defenses. The more you understand the profound role your gut plays in your immune health, the more empowered you'll feel to make the changes that will allow your body to grow.

By nurturing your gut and immune system together, you're building a foundation for long-term health, energy, and vitality. Your gut truly is the body's command center—when it's in balance, everything else falls into place.

CHAPTER 3

Gut Health and Its Connection to Chronic Illness

The idea that a balanced gut can affect the entire body is more than just a theory—it is a well-supported scientific fact. In recent years, research has shown that the health of your gut microbiome has a profound effect on the development of chronic illnesses, autoimmune diseases, and even cancer.

The delicate balance of bacteria and other microbes in your digestive system plays a key role in how your immune system works, how inflammation is regulated, and how your body reacts to disease.

An imbalanced or "dysbiotic" gut microbiome—where harmful microbes outnumber beneficial ones—can cause a cascade of problems that add to a variety of chronic conditions.

These imbalances can trigger inflammation, impair immune function, and disrupt the body's ability to handle stress and repair itself. In this chapter, we will explore how an unhealthy gut microbiome can add to autoimmune diseases, cancer, and other chronic health conditions, and most importantly, how you can take steps to restore balance to your gut to protect your health.

The Role of the Gut in Autoimmune Diseases

An autoimmune disease happens when the immune system mistakenly attacks the body's own tissues, thinking they are foreign invaders.

Diseases like rheumatoid arthritis, multiple sclerosis, lupus, and Type 1 diabetes are all examples of autoimmune diseases. But what if we told you that your gut health could play a major role in the onset of these diseases?

Research has shown that the gut microbiome has a direct impact on the immune system, and when the balance of microbes is disrupted, the immune system may become "overactive" or "misguided." This can result in the immune system attacking healthy tissue in the body, leading to inflammation and the symptoms of autoimmune illnesses.

One of the key ways through which the gut microbiome influences autoimmune diseases is through intestinal permeability, often referred to as "leaky gut." In a healthy gut, the lining of the intestines works as a barrier, allowing nutrients to pass into the bloodstream while blocking harmful substances, such as toxins and pathogens. However, in a dysbiotic gut, this barrier can weaken, leading to greater intestinal permeability.

When the gut lining is compromised, harmful bacteria and toxins can leak into the bloodstream, causing an immune response. Over time, this chronic inflammation can lead to the development of autoimmune illnesses. Conditions like rheumatoid arthritis and inflammatory bowel disease (IBD) have been strongly linked to imbalances in the gut bacteria, as dysbiosis leads to increased inflammation and immune dysfunction.

The Gut's Link to Cancer Development

Cancer is a multifactorial disease, meaning that multiple factors add to its development. One of the new factors is the gut microbiome. The microbes in your gut can influence cancer growth in several ways, including by affecting inflammation, immune function, and even how DNA is repaired. Chronic inflammation is a known risk factor for different types of cancer. In a healthy body, the immune system helps control inflammation, turning it off when it's no longer needed.

However, when the gut microbiome is out of balance, harmful bacteria can lead to ongoing low-grade inflammation throughout the body, which in turn can increase the risk of cancer.

For example, colorectal cancer has been linked to changes in the gut bacteria. Certain types of bacteria, such as those producing specific metabolites, can create an environment that supports the growth of cancer cells in the colon.

Additionally, an imbalanced microbiome may impair the immune system's ability to find and destroy cancer cells before they can proliferate. The gut also plays a major role in regulating the body's immune response to tumors. A healthy gut microbiome can stimulate the production of certain immune cells that help fight cancer, while a dysbiotic microbiome may impair this process, allowing cancer cells to avoid detection.

This is why researchers are exploring the possibility of using probiotics, prebiotics, and dietary interventions to restore gut health and reduce the risk of cancer.

Chronic Inflammation: The Root of Many Diseases

Chronic inflammation is at the heart of many modern illnesses. Conditions such as heart disease, diabetes, and obesity have all been linked to prolonged inflammation in the body, which is often the result of an unhealthy gut bacteria.

When the balance of bacteria in the gut is disrupted, it can lead to the activation of the immune system, causing an inflammatory reaction.

In a state of dysbiosis, the body's immune system stays in a heightened state of alert, constantly battling against perceived threats. This leads to systemic inflammation, which damages tissues and systems over time.

Chronic inflammation has been implicated in conditions like:

Cardiovascular disease: Inflammation plays a major role in the development of atherosclerosis (plaque buildup in the arteries) and other heart conditions.

Metabolic disorders: Chronic low-grade inflammation adds to insulin resistance, a precursor to Type 2 diabetes and obesity.

Neurodegenerative diseases: Conditions such as Alzheimer's disease and Parkinson's disease are thought to be worsened by inflammation in the brain.

Gut Imbalances and Chronic Fatigue Syndrome Another growing area of worry is the link between gut health and chronic fatigue syndrome (CFS).

Individuals with CFS often experience persistent fatigue, muscle pain, and trouble concentrating, despite getting adequate rest. While the exact cause of CFS remains unclear, new studies show that an imbalanced gut microbiome may contribute to the development of this debilitating condition.

Dysbiosis in the gut can lead to immune system dysfunction and chronic inflammation, both of which have been involved in CFS. Additionally, an unhealthy gut can affect the gut-brain axis, the communication pathway between the gut and the brain, which plays a key role in regulating mood and energy levels.

An imbalance in gut bacteria may therefore not only add to the physical symptoms of CFS but also to the cognitive and emotional symptoms.

How to Protect Your Gut and Prevent Chronic Illness

The good news is that you have the power to support your gut health and reduce your chance of developing chronic diseases by taking a proactive approach to your diet and lifestyle. Here are some methods to help you restore balance to your gut microbiome:

1. Eat a diverse, plant-based diet: A varied diet rich in fiber, fruits, veggies, whole grains, and fermented foods can nourish beneficial gut bacteria and promote a healthy microbiome.

2. Include prebiotics and probiotics: Prebiotics are foods that feed good bacteria in the gut, while probiotics are live microorganisms that can help restore balance. Foods like yogurt, kefir, cabbage, and kimchi are great sources of probiotics, while onions, garlic, and bananas are rich in prebiotics.

3. Avoid excessive use of antibiotics: While antibiotics are important for treating infections, overuse can harm the balance of bacteria in your gut. Always take antibiotics as recommended and consider discussing alternatives with your healthcare provider when possible.

4. Manage stress: Chronic stress can wreak havoc on your gut health. Practicing stress-management methods such as meditation, deep breathing, yoga, or even regular physical exercise can help regulate the gut-brain axis and reduce inflammation.

5. Limit processed foods and sugar: Processed foods, artificial sweeteners, and refined sugars can encourage the growth of dangerous bacteria and promote dysbiosis. opt for whole, nutrient-dense foods to feed your gut the energy it needs.

6. Consider gut-healing supplements: Certain supplements, like L-glutamine, zinc, and omega-3 fatty acids, can help support gut health and lower inflammation. Consult with a healthcare worker before adding any new supplements to your routine.

The connection between your gut and chronic illness is a complex, but important part of understanding your body's overall health. An imbalanced gut microbiome can add to a wide range of diseases, from autoimmune conditions to cancer and metabolic disorders.

By prioritizing gut health and choosing a balanced, nourishing lifestyle, you can help protect yourself from these chronic conditions and lead a healthier, more vibrant life.

Taking care of your gut is not just about improving digestion; it's about enhancing your body's ability to fight disease, control inflammation, and maintain overall balance. The steps you take today can lay the foundation for a healthier tomorrow.

Part 2: Gut Health in Action: Its Impact on Your Daily Life

CHAPTER 4

Intermittent Fasting: The Gut Reset

In the modern world, where we're constantly on the go, bombarded with food options, and often eating out of habit rather than hunger, we've forgotten something crucial: the power of giving our gut system a break. The idea of intermittent fasting (IF) isn't just about weight loss or a popular diet—it's about rejuvenating your gut and resetting your digestion to work more efficiently.

Intermittent fasting has gained major popularity in recent years, but its roots go far deeper than modern fads. This practice includes cycling between periods of eating and fasting, allowing the body time to repair and rejuvenate itself. Far from just a tool for weight loss, intermittent fasting has proven benefits for gut health, digestion, and general wellness.

In this chapter, we'll explore how intermittent fasting works, the science behind it, and how it can help reset your gut to promote better digestion, reduce inflammation, and improve your general health. Whether you're looking to enhance your digestive system, control your weight, or improve your energy levels, intermittent fasting can be a powerful tool in your wellness journey.

What is Intermittent Fasting?

Intermittent eating isn't about what you eat, but rather when you eat. Unlike traditional diets that focus on calorie restriction or specific food groups, intermittent fasting includes alternating periods of eating and fasting. During fasting times, the body goes into a state of repair, where it breaks down old, damaged cells and regenerates new, healthy ones.

There are various ways to implement intermittent fasting, but some of the most popular methods include:

1. The 16/8 method: This method requires fasting for 16 hours and eating within an 8-hour window. For example, you might eat between noon and 8 PM and fast from 8 PM until noon the next day.

2. The 5:2 method: In this technique, you eat normally for five days of the week and restrict calories to around 500-600 on the other two non-consecutive days.

3. Eat-Stop-Eat: This method requires fasting for a full 24 hours once or twice a week. While these are the most common methods, intermittent fasting can be tailored to fit your lifestyle. It isn't a one-size-fits-all approach; it's about finding a rhythm that works for your body and health goals.

How Intermittent Fasting Benefits Your Gut

Intermittent fasting provides your body with several unique advantages, especially when it comes to gut health. Here's how fasting can help reset your digestive system and promote general wellness:

1. Improved Digestion and Gut Rest

One of the most obvious benefits of intermittent fasting is the rest it provides for your gut. When you eat continuously, your digestive system is constantly working, breaking down food and receiving nutrients. However, giving your gut a break from this constant cycle of digestion allows your body to focus on repair and rejuvenation. During fasting periods, the gut can rest, heal, and regenerate, which is crucial for keeping healthy digestion over time.

Additionally, fasting pushes the gut lining to repair itself. This is important because an unhealthy gut lining can lead to conditions like leaky gut syndrome, where toxins and undigested food particles leak into the bloodstream, causing inflammation and possibly triggering autoimmune diseases. A time of fasting helps reinforce the integrity of the gut lining, ensuring that it functions properly.

2. Reduction of Inflammation

Chronic inflammation is a key contributor to many gut-related diseases, such as irritable bowel syndrome (IBS), Crohn's disease, and ulcerative colitis. Studies have shown that intermittent fasting can lower signs of inflammation in the body, promoting a healthier gut environment. By giving your body time to focus on reducing inflammation rather than digesting food constantly, intermittent fasting helps control the inflammation that may contribute to digestive discomfort.

3. Enhancement of Gut Microbiome Diversity

Your gut microbiome—the trillions of microorganisms living in your digestive tract—plays a vital role in digestion, immunity, and general health. Research has shown that intermittent fasting can improve the diversity of gut microbiota, which is important for a well-functioning digestive system. A diverse microbiome helps with nutrient absorption, metabolism, and protects your body against harmful bacteria or viruses. Fasting has been shown to promote the growth of beneficial bacteria, while reducing the number of harmful microbes that may disrupt gut health.

4. Promotion of Autophagy and Cellular Repair

During fasting, your body starts a process called autophagy. This is where your cells break down and remove broken components, including any dysfunctional gut cells. By promoting autophagy, intermittent fasting helps clear out old or damaged gut cells, allowing your gut to renew and regenerate with healthier cells. This cellular repair is crucial for keeping a healthy gut lining, improving digestion, and enhancing overall gut function.

5. Stabilization of Blood Sugar Levels

Elevated blood sugar levels can lead to insulin resistance, which in turn can disrupt gut health. High insulin levels are linked to an increase in gut inflammation, and an imbalance of insulin can affect the gut's ability to keep a healthy microbiome. Intermittent fasting helps maintain blood sugar levels by improving the body's sensitivity to insulin. This stabilization has a good ripple effect on gut health, preventing conditions like gut dysbiosis and metabolic syndrome that can arise from poor blood sugar regulation.

Intermittent Fasting and Your Overall Wellness

While the main focus of intermittent fasting is on your gut and digestion, the benefits go far beyond that. Many people who follow intermittent fasting experience improved mental clarity, better energy levels, and even enhanced mood. When the body is in a state of fasting, it also makes ketones, which are known to be a more efficient energy source for the brain, resulting in clearer thinking and heightened cognitive function.

Additionally, intermittent fasting has been linked to better cardiovascular health, weight management, and a reduced risk of chronic diseases like Type 2 diabetes, heart disease, and even certain types of cancer. By allowing your body to rest and reset, intermittent fasting improves not just your gut, but your entire body's ability to work optimally.

How to Get Started with Intermittent Fasting

Starting intermittent fasting may feel daunting at first, especially if you're used to eating at regular times throughout the day. However, it's important to approach it in a gradual and lasting way:

1. Start Slow

Begin with a shorter fasting window, such as 12 hours of fasting followed by 12 hours of eating. Gradually raise your fasting window over time as your body adjusts.

2. Listen to Your Body

If you feel overly fatigued or experience dizziness, it may be a sign to ease up or adjust your fasting plan. It's important to keep balance and not force your body into a fasting routine that feels uncomfortable.

3. Stay Hydrated

Drink plenty of water throughout the fasting time to stay hydrated. Herbal teas or black coffee (without sugar or cream) can also be taken during the fasting window to curb hunger.

4. Focus on Whole Foods

During your eating window, favour nutrient-dense, whole foods such as vegetables, lean proteins, healthy fats, and whole grains. Avoid overeating or bingeing, as this can counteract the benefits of fasting.

Intermittent fasting is more than just a trendy diet—it's a powerful tool for resetting your gut, promoting healthy digestion, reducing inflammation, and improving general wellness. By giving your digestive system, the time and space it needs to rest and repair, intermittent fasting supports a more balanced and efficient gut microbiome, leading to better digestion, enhanced immunity, and improved energy levels.

With the right method, intermittent fasting can be a transformative practice for your health—one that rejuvenates not only your gut but also your mind and body, helping you to feel better, more energized, and more balanced.

Whether you're looking to enhance your digestive health, lose weight, or simply optimize your general wellness, intermittent fasting offers a simple yet effective path toward a healthier, happier you.

CHAPTER 5

Gut Health and Weight Loss: A Symbiotic Relationship

When it comes to weight loss, most of us focus on traditional methods—caloric restriction, exercise routines, or trying the latest diet trend. We often forget one important player in the equation: the gut microbiome. For many years, the gut was simply considered a digestive system.

However, recent research has unveiled that your gut is far more than just a "food processor"—it is an active participant in your metabolic processes, appetite regulation, fat storage, and general weight management.

In fact, studies now show that the gut microbiome

plays a pivotal role in how we gain, lose, or keep weight. The balance of bacteria in your gut changes how your body processes food, extracts energy, and stores fat.

The gut also communicates directly with the brain, influencing not only what you crave but also how your body responds to food, exercise, and general metabolism. This chapter will cover how gut health is intricately connected to weight loss and metabolism and why improving gut health might be the key to sustainable weight loss.

The Gut Microbiome: A Complex System

Before delving into the connection between the gut and weight loss, it's important to understand what the gut microbiome is and how it works. The gut microbiome refers to the collection of trillions of microorganisms—bacteria, viruses, fungi, and other microbes—that live in your gastrointestinal (GI) tract. While bacteria often get a bad rap, not all bacteria are dangerous. In fact, most of the microbes in your gut are beneficial and important for your overall health.

Your microbiome is unique to you, like a fingerprint, and changes over time due to factors like food, lifestyle, antibiotics, and environmental exposure. In a healthy gut, a range of beneficial bacteria coexist, helping you break down food, produce important nutrients, and protect you from harmful pathogens.

However, when the balance of good and bad bacteria is disrupted, a condition known as dysbiosis can appear. Dysbiosis has been linked to a range of health issues, including weight gain, metabolic dysfunction, and inflammation.

Gut Bacteria and Weight Regulation

So how exactly does your gut affect your weight? Several mechanisms are at play, and new scientific studies have given compelling evidence that the gut microbiome is intricately involved in regulating fat storage, hunger, metabolism, and caloric expenditure.

1. Energy Harvesting from Food

Your gut bugs are responsible for breaking down the food you eat. While your body can process some foods on its own, certain complex carbohydrates (such as fiber) cannot be broken down by your digestive enzymes. That's where your gut bugs come in. Certain species of gut bacteria specialize in fermenting fiber and turning it into short-chain fatty acids (SCFAs), which can then be used as an energy source.

However, some bacteria take more energy from the same food than others. People with a higher abundance of certain bacteria, such as Firmicutes, may extract more calories from the same food than those with more Bacteroidetes, a different type of bacteria.

As a result, people with a higher percentage of Firmicutes might experience more weight gain, while people with more Bacteroidetes tend to burn more energy.

2. Hormonal Regulation and Appetite Control

The gut also plays a critical part in regulating hunger and satiety hormones. These hormones tell your brain when you're full or hungry, and they are highly influenced by the microbes in your gut. For example, ghrelin, known as the "hunger hormone," is released when the stomach is empty and signals to the brain that it's time to eat. On the other hand, leptin, the "satiety hormone," signals to the brain when you've had enough to eat.

Research has shown that a dysbiotic microbiome can interact with the production of these hormones, leading to increased feelings of hunger and overeating. In contrast, a healthy gut microbiome helps to control these hormones, promoting a balanced appetite and reducing overeating.

3. Fat Storage and Inflammation

Your gut bacteria also affect how your body stores fat. An imbalanced gut microbiome can cause low-grade inflammation, which can affect the way your body processes fat. This chronic inflammation can lead to insulin resistance, a situation where your body no longer responds effectively to insulin. As a result, glucose (sugar) is kept as fat instead of being used for energy. Insulin resistance is a big contributor to weight gain and is closely linked to obesity, type 2 diabetes, and metabolic syndrome.

Additionally, the gut bacteria can communicate with your fat cells and impact fat storage. When your microbiome is imbalanced, it can tell fat cells to store excess energy as fat, leading to weight gain. A healthy, balanced microbiome can help avoid this over-storage of fat by promoting proper nutrient absorption and fat metabolism.

4. Gut-Brain Connection and Cravings

There's a direct line of contact between your gut and your brain, often referred to as the gut-brain axis. This link goes both ways: your brain can send signals to your gut, and your gut can send signals to your brain. Some of these signals can affect how we perceive food, what we crave, and how we react to emotional eating.

The gut microbiome affects the production of neurotransmitters, such as serotonin and dopamine, which play a role in regulating mood and appetite. For instance, about 90% of serotonin, the "feel-good" neurotransmitter, is made in your gut. If your microbiome is out of balance, it can change serotonin production, leading to cravings for unhealthy foods or emotional eating.

By restoring balance to the microbiome, you can positively impact your mood, reduce cravings, and eventually make healthier food choices.

How to Improve Gut Health for Sustainable Weight Loss

Now that we've explored how gut health affects weight loss, the next question is: How can you improve your gut health to promote sustainable weight loss?

1. Focus on a Diverse, Plant-Rich Diet One of the most important ways to support your gut health is by eating a diverse range of foods, especially plant-based foods. The more variety in your diet, the more diversity your microbiome will have, which is important for a balanced and healthy gut.

Focus on foods that are high in fiber, such as fruits, veggies, whole grains, and legumes, as they feed the beneficial bacteria in your gut.

Additionally, include fermented foods like yogurt, kefir, kimchi, sauerkraut, and kombucha. These foods contain probiotics, which are live helpful bacteria that can help repopulate the gut with good microbes.

2. Avoid Overuse of Antibiotics

While antibiotics are important for treating bacterial infections, overusing them can harm your gut microbiome. Antibiotics don't just target dangerous bacteria—they also wipe out the good bacteria in your gut. This can disrupt the balance of your microbiome and lead to dysbiosis, which may contribute to weight gain and metabolic problems. Use antibiotics only when recommended by a healthcare provider and opt for natural remedies whenever possible.

3. Incorporate Intermittent Fasting

As discussed in a previous chapter, intermittent fasting (IF) is a useful tool for improving gut health and metabolism. During fasting periods, your gut has time to repair itself, lower inflammation, and regulate its microbial balance. Intermittent fasting also supports autophagy, the body's process of breaking down and eliminating damaged cells, which includes repairing cells in the gut lining.

4. Reduce Sugar and Processed Foods

Refined sugars and processed foods are not only bad for your general health—they're also detrimental to your gut. These foods support the growth of harmful bacteria and fungi in your gut, leading to dysbiosis and chronic inflammation. Instead, opt for whole, nutrient-dense foods, and limit the intake of sugary snacks and highly processed items.

5. Consider Probiotics and Prebiotics

To further support your gut health, try incorporating probiotics and prebiotics into your routine. Probiotics are live bacteria found in fermented foods or supplements, while prebiotics are types of fiber that feed the helpful bacteria in your gut. By taking both probiotics and prebiotics, you help support a thriving gut microbiome, which in turn can support weight control.

6. Manage Stress

Chronic stress can wreak havoc on your gut. Stress triggers the sympathetic nervous system, which can impair digestion and disrupt the balance of your microbiome. Practicing stress management techniques like meditation, yoga, deep breathing exercises, and getting regular physical movement can help keep your gut in balance and your weight in check.

Your gut and weight are closely connected, and taking care of your gut health can be the key to unlocking sustainable weight loss. By improving the balance of your gut microbiome, you can enhance your metabolism, regulate your appetite, reduce inflammation, and eventually achieve and keep a healthy weight.

Understanding the symbiotic link between your gut and your metabolism is the first step toward a healthier you. With the right lifestyle choices—such as eating a diverse diet, managing stress, adopting intermittent fasting, and supporting your gut with probiotics and prebiotics—you can create the basis for long-term weight loss success. It's time to give your gut the care it deserves and watch as your body changes from the inside out.

CHAPTER 6

That Gut Feeling: The Gut-Brain Connection

When we talk about gut health, most people instantly think of digestion and physical well-being. But what if we tell you that your gut doesn't just control your digestion—it also has a powerful effect on your emotions, stress levels, and even cognitive function? The science behind this link is more than just a theory; it's rooted in what is known as the gut-brain axis, a direct communication pathway between your gut and your brain.

This relationship between the gut and the brain has become a topic of growing study, and it has profound implications for both physical and mental health. It turns out that the gut and brain are in constant communication, influencing each other in ways that can affect everything from how you process feelings to your ability to think clearly, cope with stress, and even fight off illnesses.

In this chapter, we'll look into how the gut-brain connection works, how your gut affects your mood and cognitive function, and what you can do to support a healthier gut-brain relationship for better emotional and mental well-being.

The Gut-Brain Axis: A Two-Way Street

The gut-brain axis is a complex communication network that links the central nervous system (the brain and spinal cord) to the enteric nervous system (the "second brain" found in the gut). This connection is made possible by a number of mechanisms, including the vagus nerve, which is the longest cranial nerve and connects the brain directly to the gut. Through this nerve, your brain and gut share information in real-time.

In addition to the vagus nerve, the gut and brain interact through hormones, neurotransmitters, and immune system signaling molecules. For example, the gut produces over 90% of the body's serotonin, a neurotransmitter that controls mood, sleep, and appetite.

This is one of the reasons why gut health can have such a profound effect on mental health. If the gut is imbalanced, it can lead to disruptions in serotonin production, possibly adding to conditions like depression, anxiety, and sleep disturbances.

But the communication doesn't flow in only one way. While the brain can influence the gut (as anyone who's ever felt "butterflies" in their stomach before a stressful event knows), the gut also influences the brain.

This two-way street means that emotions, stress, and cognitive function can be affected by the gut microbiome's health, the presence of certain microbes, and the gut's general ability to function properly.

How the Gut Influences Your Emotions and Stress Levels

For years, we've been familiar with the saying, "I have a gut feeling," when we experience an emotional response to something. Interestingly, this saying is more grounded in fact than most people know. The gut has a significant part in how we experience and manage emotions and stress.

1. Mood Regulation and Anxiety:

As mentioned, serotonin, a neurotransmitter that helps regulate mood, is mainly produced in the gut. The gut's ability to create and release serotonin is therefore important to how we feel. In fact, research has shown that gut dysbiosis (an imbalance in gut bacteria) can lead to decreased serotonin production, which has been linked to mood disorders such as sadness and anxiety. Furthermore, disruptions in gut health have also been linked with irritable bowel syndrome (IBS), which can be exacerbated by emotional stress.

2. The Stress Response:

One of the most fascinating parts of the gut-brain connection is how stress can affect gut health and vice versa. Stress can cause gut permeability (often called "leaky gut"), allowing harmful chemicals and bacteria to leak into the bloodstream. This, in turn, can provoke an immune response, leading to inflammation and further dysbiosis, causing a vicious cycle. On the other hand, poor gut health can trigger an abnormal stress reaction, making it harder for the body to deal with emotional stress.

3. The Role of Gut Microbes in Emotional Health:

The gut microbiome is home to billions of microbes that interact with the body and impact neurotransmitter production. Certain beneficial gut bacteria, such as Lactobacillus and Bifidobacterium, are known to support the production of key neurotransmitters, including serotonin and gamma-aminobutyric acid (GABA), both of which play important roles in managing anxiety and stress. Conversely, an overgrowth of harmful bacteria, such as Firmicutes or Bacteroides, has been linked to higher amounts of stress, anxiety, and even depression.

4. The Impact of Gut Health on Cognitive

Function: Research is also showing that gut health doesn't just affect our emotional state—it also affects our cognitive skills. The gut-brain axis affects everything from memory and focus to decision-making and executive function. Imbalances in the gut bacteria have been linked to cognitive decline, neurodegenerative diseases like Alzheimer's, and even brain fog, which is a term used to describe a state of confusion, forgetfulness, and lack of clarity. Gut health seems to play a key part in regulating the brain's neuroplasticity, or its ability to form new connections and adapt to new information. Without proper microbial balance, neuroplasticity can be impaired, affecting mental sharpness and general cognitive function.

The Role of Inflammation in the Gut-Brain Connection

A key part of the gut-brain relationship is inflammation. Chronic inflammation in the gut can send harmful signals to the brain, adding to mood disorders, cognitive decline, and a heightened stress response. Here's how it works:

1. Inflammation in the Gut:

When the gut bacteria are out of balance, it can lead to intestinal inflammation, which may increase the permeability of the gut lining. This phenomenon, often called "leaky gut," allows toxins and bacteria to escape into the bloodstream, where they can cause an inflammatory response in the brain. This is thought to be a contributing factor in conditions like sadness, anxiety, and even schizophrenia.

2. Cytokines and the Brain:

Inflammation in the gut creates cytokines, which are immune system molecules that help protect the body from infection. However, when the body is in a chronic state of inflammation, elevated amounts of cytokines can make their way into the brain. This has been shown to disrupt normal brain function and is one of the reasons why people with inflammatory gut diseases like Crohn's disease or ulcerative colitis are more likely to experience anxiety and sadness.

How to Support a Healthy Gut-Brain Connection

Now that we understand the profound effect the gut can have on our emotional and cognitive health, the next question is: How can we nurture this gut-brain connection to improve our mental well-being? The good news is that there are real steps you can take to support a healthier gut and improve your emotional and cognitive health.

1. *Eat a Gut-Friendly Diet:*

A diet rich in fiber (found in fruits, vegetables, and whole grains) and fermented foods (like yogurt, kefir, kimchi, and sauerkraut) is one of the best ways to support a healthy gut microbiome. These foods provide important nutrients for beneficial gut bacteria and help to maintain a balanced microbiome, which is critical for mental and emotional health. Additionally, foods high in omega-3 fatty acids (like salmon, walnuts, and flaxseeds) and antioxidants (like berries and leafy greens) have anti-inflammatory effects that can help lower inflammation in both the gut and the brain.

2. Incorporate Probiotics and Prebiotics:

Probiotics are live bacteria that add to the population of healthy microbes in your gut, while prebiotics are non-digestible fibers that feed and support the growth of helpful bacteria. Incorporating both probiotics and prebiotics into your diet can help restore a healthy balance of gut bacteria and lower stress, anxiety, and even symptoms of depression.

3. Manage Stress:

Since the gut and brain are deeply connected, reducing stress is important for maintaining both gut and mental health. Practices like yoga, meditation, and mindfulness have been shown to lower stress hormones, promote calm, and improve gut health. Regular exercise is also key—moderate movement has been linked to improved gut microbiome diversity and better mood regulation.

4. Avoid Antibiotics and Other Disruptors:

While antibiotics can be important for treating infections, they can also disrupt the balance of your gut microbiome, sometimes leading to long-term health problems. Whenever possible, try to avoid unnecessary antibiotic use and focus on supporting your gut with natural, gut-friendly foods and lifestyle habits.

5. Sleep Well:

Quality sleep is important for both gut and brain health. Poor sleep can affect the gut microbiome, while an imbalanced microbiome can make it harder to fall and stay asleep. Aim for 7-9 hours of peaceful sleep per night to support both mental and physical health.

The gut-brain axis is a powerful and complex relationship that has a profound effect on your emotional and mental well-being. By understanding how your gut affects your mood, stress levels, and cognitive function, you can take steps to support a healthier gut microbiome and improve your overall health.

Through food, lifestyle changes, and stress management, you can support both your gut and your mind, creating a more balanced and vibrant you. The key to optimal health lies not just in what you eat, but in how you nurture the delicate link between your gut and brain.

CHAPTER 7

The Gut's Influence on Brain Development & Disorders

The connection between the gut and the brain might not seem clear at first. After all, the gut is mainly responsible for digesting food, while the brain controls cognitive function, emotions, and behavior. However, growing evidence shows that the health of your gut can have a profound impact on your brain function, development, and mental health.

In fact, the gut and brain are connected through a complex communication system known as the gut-brain axis, and new research has uncovered just how influential the microbiome in your gut is on your brain's health.

From regulating mood and emotions to influencing brain development and possibly adding to neurological disorders such as depression, anxiety, autism, and even Alzheimer's disease, the gut microbiome plays a key role in how the brain functions and develops.

This chapter will examine the effect of gut health on the brain, how an imbalanced gut microbiome can lead to mental health challenges and brain disorders, and practical steps you can take to support a healthy gut and, by extension, a healthy brain.

The Gut-Brain Axis: A Complex Communication System

The word gut-brain axis refers to the intricate system of communication between your gut and brain. This pathway allows signals to travel back and forth between these two organs, which might seem like separate systems, but are in fact, highly interconnected.

The gut-brain axis includes various communication channels, including the vagus nerve, the immune system, and chemical signals such as neurotransmitters.

1. Vagus Nerve:

The vagus nerve is one of the main communication pathways between the gut and brain. It stretches from the brainstem down to the abdomen and is responsible for carrying information about the state of your digestive system to the brain. This can include messages about satiety (feeling full), discomfort, or even emotional states caused by digestive issues.

2. Immune System:

The gut is home to a large portion of the body's immune system. When the gut microbiome is imbalanced, it can cause inflammation in the gut, which may then affect the brain. This chronic inflammation is thought to play a key role in mood disorders like sadness and anxiety.

3. Neurotransmitters and Chemical Messengers:

The gut microbiome produces a range of chemicals that are also produced in the brain. For example, around 90% of serotonin, a neurotransmitter that helps manage mood, is produced in the intestines. Other chemicals like dopamine, which affect motivation and reward pathways, are also created by gut microbes. An imbalance in these chemicals can directly impact brain health and performance.

Gut Health and Brain Development

Your gut plays an essential role in brain development, especially in the early stages of life. Emerging study has shown that the gut microbiome affects the development of the central nervous system (CNS), which includes the brain and spinal cord. A healthy gut microbiome is important for optimal brain development, as it helps to control the formation of brain circuits and the maturation of brain cells.

1. Early Life and Microbiome growth:

During infancy and early childhood, the gut microbiome undergoes rapid growth. The types of bacteria present in the gut can affect neurodevelopmental outcomes, including cognitive development, emotional regulation, and social behavior. Disruptions to the gut microbiome during this critical period of brain development, such as from antibiotic use, poor diet, or infections, have been linked with neurodevelopmental delays and behavioral problems.

2. *The Role of Gut Microbes in Neurogenesis:*

Neurogenesis is the process by which new neurons (nerve cells) are created, and it is important for learning, memory, and overall brain function. Research shows that a healthy gut microbiome plays a role in stimulating neurogenesis, especially in areas of the brain like the hippocampus, which is responsible for memory and learning. An imbalance in gut microbes can hinder neurogenesis, possibly adding to cognitive decline and learning difficulties.

Gut Health and Neurological Disorders

In addition to affecting brain development, an imbalanced gut microbiome is increasingly being linked to neurological and psychiatric disorders. This link has led researchers to explore the possibility that improving gut health could help in the treatment or prevention of conditions like depression, anxiety, autism spectrum disorder (ASD), and neurodegenerative diseases like Alzheimer's and Parkinson's.

1. Depression and Anxiety:

Research has shown that there is a strong link between the gut microbiome and mood regulation. Imbalances in the gut bacteria, often referred to as dysbiosis, can lead to inflammation that affects the brain, especially areas involved in mood regulation like the prefrontal cortex and limbic system.

a). Serotonin and the Gut: As mentioned earlier, about 90% of serotonin, the neurotransmitter responsible for mood regulation, is made in the gut. Low serotonin levels in the brain are a hallmark of sadness. Therefore, any disruptions in gut health that affect serotonin production can possibly contribute to mood disorders.

b). Inflammation and Depression: Chronic low-grade inflammation, often coming from an unhealthy gut microbiome, has been linked to depression. Inflammatory cytokines, produced by immune cells in the gut, can enter the bloodstream and affect the brain, adding to symptoms of depression and anxiety.

2. Autism Spectrum Disorder (ASD):

Emerging evidence shows that the gut microbiome may play a role in the development of autism spectrum disorder (ASD). Research has found that children with ASD tend to have unique gut microbiomes compared to neurotypical children.

Imbalances in gut bacteria may affect brain growth and behavior, leading to the social and cognitive challenges associated with ASD. Some studies have even suggested that gut dysbiosis could add to the gut-related symptoms (such as constipation or diarrhea) often seen in individuals with autism.

3. Neurodegenerative Diseases:

Alzheimer's and Parkinson's disease are neurodegenerative illnesses that lead to the progressive loss of cognitive function and motor skills. Recent study has suggested that the gut microbiome may play a role in the development of these conditions. For example, people with Alzheimer's disease often have an overgrowth of certain bacteria that contribute to inflammation in the brain, while those with Parkinson's disease have been found to have imbalances in their gut microbiome that may influence the accumulation of alpha-synuclein, a protein linked to Parkinson's. Maintaining a healthy gut microbiome could, in theory, help to lower inflammation and slow the progression of these diseases.

Supporting Gut and Brain Health

Now that we understand how the gut influences brain function and neural health, it's important to focus on how we can support both the gut and the brain. Maintaining a healthy gut microbiome is key to supporting optimal brain development and preventing or managing neurological disorders. *Here are some useful tips:*

1. Eat a Balanced, Fiber-Rich Diet:

Your diet plays a key role in shaping the health of your gut microbiome. A diet rich in fiber, especially from fruits, vegetables, and whole grains, offers food for beneficial gut bacteria. Fiber-rich foods also support the growth of prebiotics, which help feed probiotics, the beneficial bacteria that control gut health.

2. Incorporate Probiotics:

Probiotics are live bacteria and yeasts that are helpful to the gut. They can help restore balance to the gut microbiome by raising the number of healthy bacteria. Fermented foods like yogurt, kimchi, cabbage, and kefir are great sources of probiotics. Additionally, probiotic supplements may help handle dysbiosis and improve both gut and brain health.

3. Manage Stress:

Chronic stress can greatly impact gut health and, in turn, brain function. The brain and gut are closely connected through the vagus nerve, and stress can cause changes in gut microbiota that contribute to inflammation and other health problems. Engaging in relaxation techniques like yoga, meditation, and deep breathing exercises can help lower stress and support a healthy gut-brain connection.

4. Get Regular Exercise:

Regular physical exercise has been shown to improve both gut health and brain function. Exercise helps regulate the microbiome by raising the diversity of beneficial bacteria in the gut. It also improves brain function by promoting the growth of new neurons in the brain and improving mood regulation.

5. Consider Gut-Healing Supplements:

Certain supplements, such as L-glutamine, fish oil, and collagen, can help support the gut lining and lower gut inflammation. Additionally, omega-3 fatty acids, which are found in fish oil, have been shown to lower inflammation in the brain and improve mood.

The relationship between the gut and the brain is incredibly complex and multifaceted, but the study is clear: gut health plays a key role in brain development, function, and emotional well-being. Imbalances in the gut microbiome can lead to a range of neurological and psychiatric disorders, including depression, anxiety, autism, and even neurodegenerative diseases like Alzheimer's and Parkinson's.

The good news is that by supporting gut health—through a balanced diet, probiotics, stress management, exercise, and gut-healing supplements—you can nurture both your brain and gut, improving your mental health and possibly reducing the risk of neurological disorder.

CHAPTER 8

The Psychobiotic Revolution: Food, Mood, and Mental Health

It's no secret that what we eat has a direct effect on our physical health, but what if the foods we consume also influence our mental health and emotions? The connection between the food we eat and our mood is not just a passing trend—it's based in science.

Welcome to the world of psychobiotics, a revolutionary idea that explores how the gut microbiome (the bacteria and other microbes living in our gut) and the food we consume interact to shape our emotional and mental well-being.

In recent years, researchers have found fascinating links between the gut and the brain, showing that the gut microbiome doesn't just help us digest food—it also plays a major role in regulating mood, cognition, and even mental health disorders like depression, anxiety, and stress.

This chapter will dive deep into the science behind psychobiotics, how gut bacteria interact with the foods we eat to affect our mental state, and practical ways to improve your emotional and mental well-being through diet.

What Are Psychobiotics?

The word psychobiotics refers to a group of probiotics—the beneficial bacteria found in fermented foods or supplements—that have been shown to have a positive effect on mental health. The name comes from the combination of "psyche", meaning the mind or mental state, and "biotics", relating to living organisms.

Research has proven that certain strains of probiotics can affect the brain by altering the way the gut and brain communicate. In fact, the gut is often referred to as the "second brain" because of its role in producing neurotransmitters and hormones that affect mood and feelings.

It's believed that the gut microbiome makes about 90% of the body's serotonin, a neurotransmitter that plays a key role in regulating mood, sleep, and emotional responses.

These gut bacteria, in turn, are changed by the foods we eat. Just as the gut influences the brain, the foods we eat can change the composition of our microbiome. By picking foods that promote a healthy balance of beneficial gut bacteria, we can possibly improve our mood, reduce stress, and even manage symptoms of mental health conditions like depression and anxiety.

The Gut-Brain Communication: How Does It Work?

The gut and the brain are linked through the gut-brain axis, a communication system that transmits signals between the two organs. The main pathways of this connection include the vagus nerve, which runs from the brain to the gut and works as a two-way communication highway, and the immune system, which helps to modulate inflammation and other factors related to both gut and brain health.

When our gut is healthy and populated with beneficial bacteria, it can produce chemicals, such as short-chain fatty acids (SCFAs), which have been shown to affect brain function and reduce inflammation.

These SCFAs can act as neurotransmitters, helping to regulate mood and brain function. On the other hand, an imbalanced microbiome—often referred to as dysbiosis—can lead to increased inflammation, which has been linked with conditions like depression, anxiety, and cognitive decline.

In addition to affecting mood through neurotransmitter production, gut bacteria can also affect the stress response. For example, studies have shown that a healthy gut microbiome can reduce the release of cortisol, the body's stress hormone, thereby helping to control stress and anxiety levels. Conversely, an unhealthy gut may cause an overproduction of cortisol, leading to heightened anxiety and mental instability.

Food and Mental Health: What's the Link?

It's clear that the health of your gut microbiome plays a major role in your mental health, but how does food fit into this equation? The foods we eat directly impact the composition of our microbiome, which in turn influences how our brain works. Certain foods nourish good bacteria, while others may promote the growth of harmful microbes.

The better we eat, the better our gut can connect with our brain to keep us feeling calm, focused, and emotionally balanced.

Here's a closer look at how specific foods affect gut health and mental health:

1. Probiotic-Rich Foods: Building Healthy Gut Bacteria

Probiotics are live microorganisms that are beneficial to our health, especially for our gut. These "good" bacteria can help balance the gut microbiome, improve digestion, and even boost happiness. Foods like yogurt, kefir, kimchi, sauerkraut, and miso are rich in probiotics and have been linked to changes in mental health.

Research shows that lactobacilli and bifidobacteria, two popular strains of probiotics, can have a good effect on mood regulation and can help reduce symptoms of depression and anxiety. In one study, people who consumed a diet rich in fermented foods containing probiotics reported having lower levels of social anxiety and better overall mood.

Incorporating these probiotic-rich foods into your diet regularly could potentially provide significant mental health benefits, especially when combined with other healthy dietary practices.

2. Prebiotics: Feeding Your Gut Microbes

Prebiotics are foods that contain fibers and plant chemicals that feed the beneficial bacteria in the gut. They help these probiotics grow and improve the balance of your gut microbiome. Some of the best prebiotic foods include garlic, onions, asparagus, bananas, apples, beans, and artichokes.

By fueling your gut microbiome with prebiotics, you're supporting the growth of bacteria that make beneficial metabolites like short-chain fatty acids (SCFAs). These SCFAs play an important part in regulating inflammation, improving gut barrier function, and supporting mental health.

3. Omega-3 Fatty Acids: The Brain's Best Friend

Omega-3 fatty acids, found in foods like fatty fish (salmon, sardines), flaxseeds, chia seeds, and walnuts, have been shown to support brain health and improve mental well-being. They can reduce brain inflammation, improve cognitive function, and even guard against neurodegenerative diseases.

Additionally, omega-3s have a direct effect on the gut microbiome. Studies have found that these healthy fats can increase the abundance of beneficial gut bacteria, improving general gut health and possibly reducing symptoms of depression and anxiety.

4. Anti-inflammatory Foods: Reducing Brain Inflammation

Chronic inflammation is a key contributor to many mental health problems, including depression and anxiety. Inflammation in the brain can disrupt normal neurotransmission and cognitive performance, leading to mood disturbances. Fortunately, certain foods can help lower inflammation both in the gut and in the brain.

Foods that are rich in antioxidants and anti-inflammatory compounds, like berries, leafy greens, turmeric, and green tea, can help lower inflammation in the body and brain. These foods are particularly beneficial for individuals dealing with mood disorders, as they may help alleviate symptoms of depression and anxiety by lowering systemic inflammation.

5. Foods to Avoid for Better Mental Health

Just as some foods promote gut and brain health, others can have a bad effect. Highly processed foods, sugary snacks, and refined carbohydrates can contribute to an imbalance in the gut microbiome, possibly worsening mental health. These foods can increase inflammation in the body, impair gut barrier function, and lead to dysbiosis, which can be linked to mood swings, anxiety, and sadness.

Limiting your intake of sugar, refined grains, trans fats, and fake additives can help protect your gut and improve mental well-being.

Supporting Mental Health with Diet: A Holistic Approach

The field of psychobiotics is still evolving, but the study is clear: what we eat matters, not just for our physical health, but for our mental health as well. By supporting a healthy gut microbiome with a balanced diet rich in probiotics, prebiotics, omega-3 fatty acids, and anti-inflammatory foods, we can create the ideal environment for emotional well-being and mental clarity.

Incorporating these dietary changes, along with managing stress, staying physically active, and practicing mindfulness, can go a long way toward improving your mood and general mental health. Eating well is not just about losing weight or getting in shape—it's about feeding both the body and the mind.

By embracing the power of food and the psychobiotic revolution, you can take control of your mental health and begin feeling more balanced, calm, and mentally stable.

The link between food, gut health, and mental well-being is a groundbreaking area of study. What you eat can directly affect the composition of your gut microbiome, which in turn impacts your brain, emotions, and overall mental health.

By making mindful choices about the foods, you eat—foods that nourish your gut and your brain— you can unlock better emotional health, lower anxiety and depression, and support overall mental clarity. The psychobiotic revolution is here, and it's an exciting chance for all of us to take better care of our minds by first caring for our gut.

CHAPTER9.

Gut-Skin Connection: The Secret to Healthy Skin

If you've ever battled with acne, eczema, or other skin conditions, you might have thought what's causing them. While skincare products, external factors like pollution, and genetics often come to mind, there's a surprise, yet increasingly recognized, cause: your gut health.

The link between your gut and skin is not just theoretical; it's a powerful and scientifically supported relationship known as the gut-skin axis. This gut-skin link is a growing area of study, showing that the health of the gut microbiome—the collection of bacteria, viruses, and other microbes living in the digestive tract—can significantly influence the condition of your skin. Poor gut health can add to common skin problems like acne, eczema, and psoriasis, while improving gut health can lead to clearer, more vibrant skin.

In this chapter, we will explore the science behind the gut-skin axis, how gut imbalances like dysbiosis (an unhealthy gut microbiome) add to skin conditions, and how improving your gut health can help you achieve a healthier complexion.

If you've been struggling with skin problems and haven't seen results from topical treatments, it might be time to look deeper—into your gut.

Understanding the Gut-Skin Axis

The gut-skin axis is the term used to describe the relationship between the gut and the skin, which interact with each other through several mechanisms. The microbiome in your gut has a profound effect on your immune system, hormone balance, and inflammation levels—factors that are directly linked to the health of your skin.

Your gut houses billions of microorganisms, including both beneficial bacteria and possibly harmful ones. When your gut microbiome is balanced, these microbes work harmoniously to support overall health, including keeping a healthy complexion. However, when the gut microbiome becomes imbalanced—a disease called dysbiosis— it can lead to systemic inflammation and skin problems. Let's break down how this link works.

The Role of Inflammation in Skin Health

One of the most important ways that the gut microbiome affects skin health is through inflammation. Inflammation is a natural process that happens when the body's immune system responds to injury or infection. However, chronic inflammation—which can come from an imbalance in the gut microbiome—can negatively impact the skin.

Conditions like acne, eczema, psoriasis, and rosacea are often linked to inflammation, and an unhealthy gut can cause or worsen these inflammatory conditions. Dysbiosis (imbalance in the gut's bacteria) can lead to an overactive immune reaction, causing inflammation that affects not only the gut but the skin as well. When the body is in a state of inflammation, the skin's barrier function becomes weakened, leading to a host of skin problems, including acne flare-ups, dryness, redness, and irritation.

By keeping a balanced gut microbiome, you can reduce chronic inflammation, which in turn can help prevent or alleviate many skin conditions. In fact, probiotics, which are beneficial bacteria found in fermented foods and supplements, can help balance the gut microbiome and, as a result, lower inflammation throughout the body, including the skin.

The Immune System and Skin Health

Around 70-80% of the body's immune system lives in the gut. This means that the gut microbiome has a direct impact on the body's immune responses, including how the immune system interacts with the skin. When the gut microbiome is disrupted, it can lead to immune dysfunction, leading the immune system to become overactive or underactive. This immune imbalance can lead to skin conditions like eczema, acne, rosacea, and even conditions like psoriasis.

A balanced gut microbiome, on the other hand, helps regulate the immune system and avoids an overactive immune response. By improving gut health through dietary changes or the use of probiotics, you can support immune balance, reducing the chance of inflammation and skin flare-ups.

Gut Bacteria and Hormonal Balance

Your gut also plays a major role in hormonal balance—especially hormones that affect the skin. Hormones such as cortisol, insulin, and androgens can all impact the skin. For instance, elevated levels of cortisol, the stress hormone, can lead to increased oil production in the skin, which can add to acne. Hormonal imbalances are also a known trigger for conditions like polycystic ovary syndrome (PCOS), which often results in acne and other skin problems.

A healthy gut microbiome helps manage hormone production by controlling inflammation and influencing the production of certain hormones. If your gut is imbalanced, it can lead to hormonal changes that negatively impact the skin. By focusing on gut health, you can help balance hormone levels, which can, in turn, improve skin health and reduce acne, oiliness, and other hormonal skin problems.

How Gut Health Affects Acne and Other Skin Conditions

Acne is one of the most common skin conditions linked to an imbalanced gut microbiome. When the gut is inflamed, it produces higher amounts of cytokines, which are inflammatory molecules that can exacerbate skin conditions like acne.

Moreover, dysbiosis in the gut has been linked to increased levels of androgens, which are hormones that can increase oil production in the skin and add to clogged pores and acne.

Eczema, another common skin disease, is also closely linked to gut health. Eczema is often caused by an overactive immune system, which is affected by the gut microbiome. Research has found that people with eczema tend to have an imbalanced gut microbiome, with fewer beneficial bacteria and more harmful ones. By restoring balance in the gut, it's possible to reduce the severity of eczema flare-ups and improve the health of the skin.

For people with psoriasis, a chronic autoimmune condition that causes skin cells to multiply too quickly, gut health can also play a major role. Studies have shown that people with psoriasis often have a disrupted gut microbiome, and improving gut health through diet or probiotics has been shown to reduce symptoms.

How to Improve Gut Health for Better Skin

Now that we understand the connection between gut health and skin health, the next question is: How can we improve our gut health to help our skin? Here are several steps you can take:

1. Eat a Gut-Friendly Diet

A healthy, well-balanced diet rich in fiber, prebiotics, and probiotics can help nourish your gut microbiome and lower inflammation.

- Prebiotics, found in foods like garlic, onions, leeks, and bananas, feed the helpful bacteria in your gut.
- Probiotics, found in fermented foods like yogurt, kefir, sauerkraut, and kimchi, bring new healthy bacteria into your gut.

Additionally, focus on eating whole, unprocessed foods while reducing your intake of sugar, refined carbs, and processed foods, which can promote dysbiosis and inflammation.

2. Take Probiotic Supplements

Probiotics are beneficial bacteria that can help reset the balance of your gut microbiome. Supplementing with probiotics can help lower inflammation, improve the immune response, and support overall gut health. This can have a positive effect on skin health, especially for conditions like acne, eczema, and psoriasis.

3. Manage Stress

Stress has a significant effect on both gut health and skin health. It can lead to hormonal imbalances, increased inflammation, and flare-ups of skin diseases like acne and eczema. Managing stress through techniques like yoga, meditation, and deep breathing can improve both gut and skin health.

4. Stay Hydrated

Drinking plenty of water is important for both gut health and skin health. Proper hydration helps flush out toxins from the body, lowers the look of dryness and wrinkles, and supports the balance of gut bacteria.

The gut-skin connection is an exciting area of study that is revealing just how important our gut health is for maintaining a clear, vibrant complexion. A balanced gut microbiome plays a key role in regulating inflammation, supporting immune function, and balancing hormones—all factors that directly impact the health of our skin.

By focusing on better gut health through a nutrient-rich diet, probiotics, and stress management, we can not only improve our digestion but also support clear, glowing skin.

So, if you've been struggling with skin issues despite using different skincare products, it might be time to take a closer look at your gut. A better gut could be the secret to unlocking healthier, more radiant skin from the inside out.

Part 3: Personalizing Your Gut Health Journey

CHAPTER 10

Prebiotics & Probiotics: The Building Blocks of Gut Health

When we talk about gut health, we often hear words like prebiotics and probiotics. These two elements are critical in restoring and keeping a healthy gut microbiome, which plays a fundamental role in overall health. In recent years, scientific research has highlighted the importance of keeping the right balance of prebiotics and probiotics to support digestion, immune function, mental health, and even skin conditions.

In this chapter, we'll dive deep into what prebiotics and probiotics are, how they work, and how they can help restore the delicate balance of your gut microbiome. With a focus on practical, science-backed information, we'll also explore how you can integrate these elements into your daily diet to optimize your gut health and improve your general well-being.

What Are Prebiotics?

Prebiotics are naturally occurring, non-digestible food components that promote the growth and action of beneficial bacteria in the gut. Essentially, prebiotics are the "food" for probiotics—the good bacteria that live in your digestive system.

Prebiotics are usually a form of fiber or complex carbohydrates that pass through the stomach and small intestine without being digested. When they reach the large intestine (or colon), they become food for the beneficial bacteria that inhabit this part of the gut.

How Do Prebiotics Work?

Once prebiotics reach the colon, they are fermented by the gut microbiota (the population of microbes living in your digestive tract), especially by the beneficial species of Bifidobacteria and Lactobacilli. This fermentation process creates short-chain fatty acids (SCFAs), such as butyrate, acetate, and propionate, which have numerous health benefits:

a). Butyrate, for example, is particularly important for the health of the cells that line your gut, as it serves as their main energy source. It has also been shown to have anti-inflammatory properties and may reduce the risk of inflammatory bowel diseases (IBD) such as Crohn's disease and ulcerative colitis.

b). SCFAs help maintain the intestinal barrier function, preventing harmful pathogens from entering the bloodstream and causing infections or inflammation.

c). They also play a role in regulating immune responses, and new research suggests they may help protect against conditions like obesity, type 2 diabetes, and even cancer.

The main function of prebiotics is to increase the growth and activity of beneficial bacteria in the gut, which, in turn, supports overall gut health and strengthens the immune system.

Prebiotic-Rich Foods

There are several food sources rich in prebiotics that can help support a healthy gut microbiome.

Some of these include:

- ***Garlic:*** Contains a substance called inulin, a type of prebiotic fiber that supports the growth of good bacteria.

- ***Onions:*** Like garlic, onions are high in inulin and also contain other prebiotic fibers.

- ***Bananas:*** Bananas are a great source of resistant starch, which works as a prebiotic. As bananas ripen, the starch content breaks down into simpler sugars that feed the good bugs in your gut.

- ***Asparagus:*** This vegetable is packed with inulin and other prebiotic fibers that help feed beneficial gut bugs.

- ***Oats:*** Rich in beta-glucans, a type of soluble fiber that serves as a prebiotic, oats support gut health and promote good bacteria growth.
- ***Apples:*** Apples contain pectin, a form of fiber that has prebiotic qualities. It helps feed healthy bacteria, especially in the colon.

By incorporating more prebiotic-rich foods into your diet, you can easily encourage the growth of beneficial bacteria in your gut, improving digestion and overall gut health.

What Are Probiotics?

Probiotics are live microorganisms that, when consumed in adequate amounts, give health benefits to the host (that's you!). These good bacteria help keep the balance of the gut microbiome by promoting the growth of beneficial bacteria and suppressing the growth of harmful bacteria and pathogens.

The most widely known strains of probiotics are Lactobacilli and Bifidobacteria, but there are many others, such as Saccharomyces boulardii (a type of yeast), Streptococcus thermophilus, and Enterococcus faecium. Probiotics can be found in soured foods, as well as in supplement form.

How Do Probiotics Work?

Probiotics work by helping to balance the bacteria environment in the gut. They provide several key benefits:

a). Supporting Digestion: Probiotics help break down food, especially in the small intestine, and can improve the absorption of nutrients. They may also help ease symptoms of irritable bowel syndrome (IBS), such as bloating, cramping, and diarrhea.

b). Boosting Immune Function: Probiotics play a key role in controlling the immune system by supporting the intestinal barrier function. A balanced microbiome stops harmful bacteria from penetrating the gut lining, reducing the risk of infections and chronic inflammation.

c). Mental Health Benefits: The gut and brain are linked via the gut-brain axis, and keeping a healthy microbiome can influence mood and stress levels. Probiotics have been shown to have a positive effect on mental health, potentially alleviating symptoms of depression, anxiety, and stress.

d). Preventing Harmful Pathogens: By promoting the growth of helpful bacteria, probiotics help create an environment that suppresses the growth of harmful bacteria and other pathogens that can cause gastrointestinal distress or infections.

Probiotic-Rich Foods

To reap the benefits of probiotics, you can eat foods that naturally contain these beneficial bacteria. Here are some popular probiotic-rich foods:

- ***Yogurt:*** One of the most popular sources of probiotics, yogurt contains live bacterial cultures that can support gut health.

- ***Kefir:*** A fermented dairy product similar to yogurt, kefir includes a wider variety of probiotic strains and is known for its ability to improve gut health and digestion.

- ***Sauerkraut:*** This fermented cabbage dish is rich in probiotics, especially Lactobacillus species, which support digestive health.

- ***Kimchi:*** A spicy Korean dish made from fermented vegetables; kimchi contains various strains of beneficial bacteria that can improve gut flora.

- ***Miso:*** A fermented soybean pastes widely used in Japanese cuisine, miso is rich in probiotics and can help maintain a healthy gut.

- ***Pickles:*** Naturally fermented pickles are another great source of probiotics, but be mindful of store-bought pickles that may contain vinegar, which doesn't encourage fermentation.

- ***Tempeh:*** Made from fermented soybeans, tempeh is not only a great source of probiotics but also rich in protein and fiber.

The Balance Between Prebiotics and Probiotics

While prebiotics and probiotics have individual benefits, their effects are greatly enhanced when taken together. Think of prebiotics as the food that helps probiotics grow. Without prebiotics, probiotics may not live or thrive in your gut. That's why a balanced diet that includes both prebiotics and probiotics is key to keeping a healthy gut microbiome.

A healthy gut bacteria supports better digestion, a stronger immune system, improved mental health, and better absorption of nutrients. The combined action of prebiotics and probiotics can help avoid gut imbalances (such as dysbiosis), which may lead to digestive disorders, weakened immunity, and even mood disorders.

How to Incorporate Prebiotics and Probiotics Into Your Diet

To take advantage of the benefits of prebiotics and probiotics, try to include a variety of these foods in your daily meals. For instance:

- Start your day with a bowl of oatmeal (prebiotic) topped with yogurt (probiotic).
- Add garlic, onions, and asparagus (prebiotics) to your salads or stir-fries.
- Enjoy kimchi or cabbage (probiotics) as a side dish with your lunch.
- Drink a glass of yoghurt or add a spoonful of miso to your soup in the evening.

In addition to food sources, prebiotics and probiotics are available in pill form, which can help ensure you're getting the right amounts of both. If you're considering supplements, speak with a healthcare provider to find the best type and dosage for your needs.

The balance between prebiotics and probiotics is important for maintaining a healthy gut microbiome. By feeding the good bacteria in your gut with prebiotics and replenishing those bacteria with probiotics, you create a gut environment that supports general health. A healthy gut can improve digestion, enhance immune function, support mental health, and even help with skin problems.

By incorporating prebiotic and probiotic-rich foods into your diet, you can take proactive steps toward optimizing your gut health and improving your general well-being.

CHAPTER 11

The Social and Environmental Factors Affecting Your Gut

Gut health is often thought to be mainly about diet—what you eat, how much you eat, and when you eat. While these factors are clearly important, the state of your gut microbiome isn't determined by food alone.

Increasingly, research has shown that lifestyle, environmental influences, and social interactions play a major role in shaping the balance of bacteria in your gut and, consequently, your overall health.

These external factors can influence everything from your digestion and defense to your mental health and even your risk for chronic diseases.

In this chapter, we'll explore how lifestyle choices, environmental factors, and social interactions affect the health of your gut. We'll also talk how you can create a gut-friendly environment by making small but impactful changes in your daily life. By knowing these external influences, you can take charge of your gut health and ensure it thrives, adding to your overall well-being.

Lifestyle Factors That Affect Your Gut Health

Your daily habits and routines are crucial in keeping or disrupting the delicate balance of your gut microbiome. Many parts of your lifestyle, from your sleep patterns to your stress levels, can impact the diversity and activity of the microorganisms in your gut.

1. Diet and Nutrition

While we've already covered the importance of food in previous chapters, it's worth reiterating that your diet is a key lifestyle factor affecting your gut. A diet rich in fiber, fermented foods, and prebiotics supports the growth of helpful bacteria.

On the other hand, a high-sugar, processed food-heavy diet can support the growth of harmful bacteria and reduce the diversity of your microbiome. The bacteria in your gut feed on the food you eat, and a healthy, balanced diet encourages the thriving of beneficial bacteria, improving both gut health and overall health.

2. Physical Activity

Exercise is another lifestyle factor that plays a pivotal role in keeping a healthy gut microbiome. Studies have shown that regular physical activity can improve the diversity of gut bacteria, which is considered a sign of a healthy microbiome. Moderate exercise, like walking, swimming, or cycling, has been shown to support beneficial bacteria such as Bacteroides, which help break down fiber and make short-chain fatty acids that have anti-inflammatory effects.

However, excessive physical activity, especially in the form of hard endurance exercise, can have the opposite effect. It can lead to gut permeability (leaky gut) and an imbalance of the microbiome, causing inflammation. It's important to find the right balance of exercise to support gut health without overtaxing the body.

3. Sleep Patterns

Adequate sleep is often overlooked when talking gut health, but the relationship between sleep and gut microbiota is strong. Studies have shown that poor sleep or irregular sleep patterns can disrupt the balance of your gut microbiome, leading to an overgrowth of harmful bacteria and a decrease in beneficial ones. Additionally, insufficient sleep can increase gut permeability, adding to inflammation and digestive issues.

A regular sleep routine with 7-9 hours of quality sleep each night supports the healthy balance of bacteria in the gut, which in turn can positively affect other aspects of your health, such as mood, energy, and immune function.

4. Stress Management

Chronic stress is one of the most important lifestyle factors that can disrupt gut health. When you're stressed, your body releases cortisol, the stress hormone, which can badly impact your microbiome. High cortisol levels can reduce the diversity of gut bacteria and lead to an imbalance that may contribute to digestive issues, inflammatory bowel diseases, and even mental health disorders like anxiety and sadness.

Practices like mindfulness, yoga, and meditation, as well as ensuring adequate rest and relaxation, are essential for managing stress and keeping a healthy gut. Reducing stress not only supports your gut but also improves your overall well-being.

Environmental Factors That Affect Your Gut Health

Your environment—the physical world around you—can greatly impact the health of your gut microbiome. While you can't control every aspect of your environment, knowing how certain factors influence your gut can help you make healthier choices and create a more gut-friendly environment.

1. Exposure to Toxins

Environmental toxins, such as pesticides, pollution, and chemicals in cleaning products, food packaging, and even personal care items, can upset your gut bacteria. These toxins can hurt the beneficial bacteria in your gut, leading to dysbiosis (an imbalance of the microbiome) and gut inflammation. Over time, this can affect your immune system, metabolism, and even your mood and mental health.

To reduce toxin exposure, you can take steps like opting for organic foods when possible, using natural cleaning and personal care products, and ensuring your home is well-ventilated to lessen indoor air pollution.

2. Antimicrobial Overuse

Antibiotics and other antimicrobial treatments are lifesaving in many cases, but they can also harm the gut microbiome when used too frequently or needlessly. Antibiotics kill both harmful and helpful bacteria, disrupting the balance of the microbiome. This disruption can lead to long-term digestive problems, immune dysfunction, and even greater susceptibility to infections.

If you need antibiotics, always follow your healthcare provider's directions and ask for probiotics or fermented foods to help restore balance to your microbiome afterward. Additionally, limiting the use of antimicrobial goods in the home, like antibacterial soaps, can help protect your gut from unnecessary disruption.

3. Urban vs. Rural Living

Where you live can also have an effect on your gut health. Studies have found that people living in more rural areas tend to have more diverse microbiomes compared to those in urban settings. This is likely due to differences in diet, lifestyle, and exposure to outdoors.

People in rural areas are more likely to be exposed to a variety of microbes from farming, animals, and natural environments, which can increase the diversity of gut bacteria.

On the other hand, urban living can subject you to higher levels of pollution, processed foods, and more sedentary lifestyles, all of which can negatively affect your gut health. If you live in a city, finding ways to incorporate outdoor activities, natural foods, and exposure to nature can help offset some of the negative effects of urban life on your gut.

Social Interactions and Their Impact on Gut Health

In addition to lifestyle and environmental factors, your social interactions can also affect the health of your gut. While it may seem unrelated at first, good social connections can have a direct effect on your gut microbiome.

1. The Importance of Socializing

Studies have shown that people who have strong social networks and regularly engage in important social interactions tend to have a more diverse gut microbiome. Socializing, particularly in positive, supportive environments, can help lower stress levels, improve feelings of happiness, and promote a healthy gut.

On the flip side, social isolation, chronic loneliness, and lack of social support have been linked to poor gut health, especially a reduction in microbial diversity. The emotional and physiological effects of loneliness can disrupt gut function and add to gut inflammation.

2. Impact of Relationships and Family Life

Our relationships with family members and close friends can also shape our gut health. Healthy, loving relationships promote a sense of emotional well-being, which can positively impact the microbiome. Children raised in homes with supportive family structures may produce healthier microbiomes, as stress is minimized and dietary habits are more stable.

Conversely, chronic stress in relationships, including family conflicts, can lead to an imbalance in the gut microbiome, just as job stress or relationship strain can.

Creating a Gut-Friendly Environment

Understanding the environmental, lifestyle, and social factors that affect your gut health is only the first step. Now that you know what can negatively affect your gut, it's time to consider how you can make a gut-friendly environment. Here are some useful tips:

1. Adopt a Gut-Healthy Diet: Focus on a diet rich in fiber, fermented foods, and prebiotics to support the growth of healthy gut bacteria. Avoid excessive processed foods and sugar, which can upset the balance of your microbiome.

2. Get Regular Exercise: Aim for moderate, consistent physical exercise, like walking, swimming, or yoga, to support a diverse microbiome. Avoid overexertion, which can harm your gut health.

3. *Manage Stress:* Practice mindfulness, meditation, and deep-breathing exercises to decrease stress levels. Adequate rest and relaxation also support a healthy gut.

4. *Prioritize Sleep:* Ensure you get 7-9 hours of quality sleep each night to help your body and gut to repair and rejuvenate.

5. *Limit Toxin Exposure:* Reduce the use of harsh chemicals, pesticides, and antimicrobial products to protect your gut microbiome from needless damage.

6. *Foster Positive Social Connections:* Build strong relationships, spend time with loved ones, and make time for social events that bring you joy.

By making small, consistent changes in these areas, you can create a gut-friendly setting that will help optimize your health and well-being. After all, a healthy gut is the basis for a healthy body and mind.

Your gut is much more than just a digestive system—it's a powerful, intricate ecosystem that influences many parts of your overall health. By knowing the social and environmental factors that affect your gut microbiome, you can take proactive steps to support its balance and function.

CHAPTER 12.

Tailoring Gut Health to You: Personalized Approaches

Gut health is often viewed through a general lens, with many articles and guides offering "one-size-fits-all" solutions. However, the truth is that each person's gut microbiome is unique, shaped by a variety of factors like genetics, food, lifestyle, and even environment.

While there are universal principles for keeping good gut health, there is no single diet, routine, or supplement that works for everyone. The key to getting optimal gut health lies in personalization—finding the strategies and practices that best support your unique microbiome.

In this chapter, we'll explore the idea of personalized gut health. We'll look at how different people respond to the same foods, diets, and supplements, and why it's important to take an individualized approach to keeping gut health. From knowing your body's specific needs to incorporating gut-friendly habits that are tailored to you, this chapter will help guide you toward a personalized path to a healthier gut and improved overall well-being.

Understanding Your Unique Gut Microbiome

The gut microbiome is an incredibly complex ecosystem of bacteria, viruses, fungi, and other microorganisms that live in your digestive tract. These microorganisms are affected by a number of factors, including:

1. Genetics: Your genetic makeup plays a role in shaping the variety and composition of your gut microbiome. Research has shown that different individuals have distinct microbial populations based on their inherited genetic traits, making some people more predisposed to specific gut-related problems like IBS or inflammatory bowel diseases.

2. Diet: What you eat can greatly impact the balance of bacteria in your gut. However, the types of foods that are beneficial for one person's microbiome may not have the same benefits on another person's gut. For example, someone with a sensitivity to dairy or gluten might experience inflammation or discomfort if they consume foods containing those ingredients, while others may have no problems.

3. *Lifestyle Choices:* Your daily habits—such as exercise, sleep, stress management, and even your social interactions—play an integral role in keeping a balanced gut. People who handle stress better or have consistent sleep patterns tend to have more diverse gut microbiomes, which are linked to better overall health.

4. *Environmental Factors:* Exposure to environmental pollutants, toxins, or even different temperatures can affect your gut health. The balance of good and bad bacteria in your gut can be swayed by the environment you live in, including things like air quality and the use of antibiotics.

Given the many factors that shape your unique microbiome, it's clear that a personalized approach to gut health is important. What works for one person may not work for another—and what improves one individual's digestion or mental health might not give the same results for someone else.

Personalized Nutrition for Gut Health

When it comes to gut health, diet plays a central part. However, finding the right foods for your unique microbiome takes some experimentation and understanding of how different foods affect your body.

1. Identifying Your Food Sensitivities

One of the first steps in tailoring your diet to support your gut health is finding any food sensitivities or intolerances you might have. Common causes for gut discomfort include:

- **Gluten:** Found in wheat, barley, and rye, gluten can be problematic for some people, especially those with celiac disease or non-celiac gluten sensitivity. For these individuals, avoiding gluten is important to maintaining gut health.

- **Dairy:** Lactose intolerance is widespread, and consuming dairy products can lead to bloating, diarrhea, or abdominal pain in sensitive people. If dairy is a problem for you, you might want to try with non-dairy alternatives like almond, oat, or coconut milk.

- **FODMAPs:** Fermentable oligosaccharides, disaccharides, monosaccharides, and polyols (FODMAPs) are a group of short-chain carbohydrates that can cause digestive pain in people with irritable bowel syndrome (IBS) or other gut conditions. Reducing high-FODMAP foods like beans, onions, and garlic may improve gut symptoms for some people.

Tracking your diet and symptoms in a food journal can help you pinpoint which foods work best for your gut and which might be causing discomfort. Additionally, working with a nutritionist or functional medicine practitioner can be helpful for identifying sensitivities and customizing your nutrition plan.

2. The Importance of Fiber and Prebiotics

Prebiotics, the non-digestible fibers in certain foods, work as food for the good bacteria in your gut. A personalized approach to prebiotics would involve focusing on the specific types of fiber that your body responds well to. Common prebiotic-rich foods include:

- *Bananas:* Rich in resistant starch, bananas are a great prebiotic food that can promote the growth of healthy gut bacteria.

- ***Garlic, onions, and leeks:*** These contain inulin, a type of prebiotic fiber that feeds beneficial bacteria.

- ***Asparagus and artichokes:*** These veggies are high in inulin and other prebiotic fibers that help nourish the gut.

Some people may find they have sensitivities to certain types of fiber. For instance, if you have IBS, you might find high-fiber foods to be tough to tolerate. In such cases, focusing on soluble fiber (which is gentler on the digestive system) rather than insoluble fiber may be helpful.

3. Probiotics: Tailoring the Right Strains to Your Needs

Probiotics are live helpful bacteria that can improve the balance of the gut microbiome. However, not all probiotics are made equal, and different strains have different effects on the body. A personalized method includes selecting the right strains based on your specific health goals.

- Lactobacillus and Bifidobacterium strains are often helpful for improving gut health and immune function.
- Saccharomyces boulardii, a type of yeast, is a probiotic strain known to help gut recovery following antibiotic treatment.
- For people with IBS, probiotics like Lactobacillus acidophilus may help alleviate symptoms like bloating and gas.

If you're unsure which probiotic strains are best for you, consider starting with a broad-spectrum probiotic that includes multiple strains, or speak with a healthcare provider to guide you toward the best choice.

Lifestyle Habits for Supporting Your Gut Microbiome

In addition to diet, your daily habits play an important part in maintaining a healthy gut. Personalized approaches to exercise, stress control, and sleep can all help optimize your gut health.

1. Exercise: Moving Your Microbes

Exercise is beneficial for your overall health, but it also has a direct effect on your gut microbiome. Regular physical exercise increases the diversity of bacteria in your gut, which is linked to better health outcomes.

While intense exercise might cause temporary changes in the microbiome (such as increased inflammation or a shift in bacterial diversity), moderate, consistent activity—like walking, cycling, or yoga—supports the growth of beneficial bacteria and improves overall gut health. The key is to find a type of exercise you enjoy and can keep regularly.

2. Stress Management

Chronic stress can negatively impact your gut microbiome by disrupting the balance of bacteria, increasing gut permeability (which may lead to leaky gut syndrome), and boosting inflammation. Personalized approaches to stress management could include practices such as:

- Mindfulness meditation
- Deep breathing exercises
- Regular physical activity (as stated above)
- Yoga or tai chi

Taking time each day to participate in stress-reducing activities can help protect your gut and ensure it remains in optimal balance.

3. Sleep Hygiene

Good quality sleep is important for maintaining a healthy microbiome. Sleep deprivation has been shown to change the gut microbiome and lower its diversity, which can negatively affect both digestion and immune function. Tailoring your sleep routine includes setting a consistent sleep schedule and ensuring your sleep environment is conducive to restful sleep.

Aim for 7-9 hours of sleep each night, and practice good sleep hygiene by reducing blue light exposure before bed and keeping a cool, quiet sleep space.

The Future of Personalized Gut Health

As we continue to learn more about the gut microbiome, personalized methods to gut health are becoming more refined. Advances in microbiome testing, genetic analysis, and nutritional science will make it easier for people to tailor their gut health strategies based on their unique needs.

Personalized medicine is changing, and it's clear that one-size-fits-all approaches to gut health are a thing of the past. By knowing your body's specific needs and making intentional changes to your diet, lifestyle, and environment, you can help support your microbiome in a way that works best for you.

Personalizing your approach to gut health is about recognizing that there is no one-size-fits-all answer. By knowing how your unique microbiome responds to different foods, habits, and lifestyle choices, you can tailor your daily routines and diet to support a healthy gut, optimize digestion, boost immunity, and improve overall well-being. It's about finding what works for your body and making lasting, long-term changes that promote balance and health.

The future of gut health is personalized, and by taking charge of your own gut health, you can achieve better results and a stronger connection between your gut and overall health.

Conclusion

The Future of Gut Health

The field of gut health is experiencing a rapid evolution. What was once considered a niche area of study has now become a major focus of medical research, with breakthroughs happening almost daily. From new scientific discoveries to cutting-edge treatments, the future of gut health holds exciting promise for improving not just digestion but general health, mental well-being, and even longevity.

In this conclusion, we will explore the latest scientific breakthroughs and emerging treatments that are shaping the future of gut health. We'll look at some of the most hopeful trends and innovations, from microbiome research and personalized medicine to novel therapies aimed at healing gut imbalances. Understanding these developments will help you stay ahead of the curve when it comes to keeping your gut health and embracing the future of wellness.

1. Microbiome Sequencing and Precision Medicine

One of the most important advances in gut health is the rise of microbiome sequencing, a technology that allows scientists to map out the composition of the microorganisms living in your gut. This process goes beyond traditional testing by identifying the specific strains of bacteria and other microbes in your gut, giving a clear picture of its general health and diversity.

In the past, many gut-related conditions like IBS (irritable bowel syndrome), Crohn's disease, and gut dysbiosis (imbalance in gut microbiota) were identified based on symptoms alone, without an understanding of the underlying microbial imbalances. However, with the rise of microbiome sequencing, doctors and researchers can pinpoint the exact microbial deficiencies or overgrowths that may be contributing to these conditions.

Precision medicine—an approach that tailors medical treatment to the individual—will soon become more available for gut health. By identifying the unique composition of a person's microbiome, healthcare providers will be able to offer personalized suggestions on diet, supplements, and probiotics that are most likely to benefit that individual.

What's Next? As microbiome sequencing technology improves and becomes more widely available, it's expected that personalized gut health solutions will become normal. Individuals may have access to tailored gut health plans based on their individual microbial makeup, leading to more effective treatments for digestive disorders, autoimmune diseases, and mental health issues linked to gut health.

2. The Rise of Psychobiotics and Mental Health Treatments

One of the most fascinating and emerging areas of gut health study is the relationship between the gut microbiome and mental health. In recent years, the field of psychobiotics has gained traction, with researchers studying how beneficial bacteria can affect brain function, mood regulation, and mental well-being. Psychobiotics are probiotics that have been shown to affect the brain, either by producing neurotransmitters like serotonin or by modulating the gut-brain axis.

In particular, the gut's role in depression, anxiety, and stress is becoming more obvious. Studies are showing that a healthy gut microbiome can support emotional regulation, reduce the effect of chronic stress, and help prevent or manage mood disorders.

The idea that we can influence our mood and mental health through our gut health is a groundbreaking concept that has deep implications for treating mental health problems.

What's Next? In the future, psychobiotics could play an important role in treating depression and anxiety. Instead of depending solely on medication, which can have side effects and may not be effective for everyone, individuals may be able to use targeted probiotics to promote mental wellness. Research into specific strains of bacteria that influence neurotransmitters and brain function is likely to increase, leading to more targeted and effective treatments for mood disorders.

3. Fecal Microbiota Transplantation (FMT) and its Potential

Another cutting-edge innovation is fecal microbiota transplantation (FMT), which includes transferring fecal matter from a healthy donor into the gut of a person with an imbalance in their microbiome. The goal is to restore a healthy balance of bacteria in the recipient's gut, and FMT has shown remarkable success in treating certain gut-related conditions, especially Clostridium difficile infections, a life-threatening bacterial infection that disrupts the gut microbiome.

FMT has already been cleared for certain uses in the treatment of C. difficile infections and is currently being studied for other gut conditions like ulcerative colitis, Crohn's disease, and even irritable bowel syndrome (IBS). Researchers are also exploring its potential in treating conditions outside of the digestive system, such as Parkinson's disease, autism spectrum disorders, and even mental health.

What's Next? As FMT research improves, it may become a viable option for people with chronic conditions that are resistant to traditional treatments. Additionally, FMT may open the door for designer microbiomes, where doctors could create custom microbiota transplants for people based on their unique microbiome profiles.

4. The Future of Probiotics: Beyond the Basics

Probiotics have been a key focus in gut health for years, and their role in supporting a healthy microbiome is well-established. However, the future of probiotics is much more than just taking a daily pill. Strain-specific probiotics are emerging as a key focus of research, with scientists working to identify specific strains that can have a therapeutic effect on different health conditions.

In the past, probiotic supplements have been marketed as a general solution to improve gut health, but the next wave of research is looking at how specific strains of Lactobacillus, Bifidobacterium, and other beneficial bacteria can be used to treat conditions like IBS, IBD (inflammatory bowel disease), and allergies, as well as mental health conditions like anxiety and depression.

What's Next? In the future, probiotic treatments may become much more personalized and targeted. People may be able to receive custom probiotics based on their gut microbiome, addressing particular health concerns and optimizing the balance of microorganisms in their digestive tract. This personalized approach to probiotics will likely transform the way we think about gut health and its effect on overall wellness.

5. New Approaches to Diet and Gut Health: From Microbial-Based Foods to Personalized Nutrition

While food has always been a cornerstone of gut health, the future of nutrition for gut health is taking a more personalized approach. Researchers are now developing microbial-based foods, which are foods especially made to nourish beneficial bacteria in the gut and improve microbiome health.

Additionally, personalized nutrition is getting ground, where diet plans are tailored to a person's unique microbiome profile. This approach takes into account factors like genetics, lifestyle, and gut composition, giving a more individualized and scientifically backed approach to gut health.

What's Next? The future of diet and nutrition for gut health will involve more precision diets, taking into account your unique gut microbiome and tailoring advice accordingly. This could mean making personalized meal plans, recommending specific prebiotics and probiotics, and optimizing nutrition based on your individual gut needs.

As we look to the future, it's clear that the field of gut health is on the brink of exciting changes. From microbiome sequencing and precision medicine to psychobiotics and fecal microbiota transplantation, the scientific community is unlocking new ways to tap the power of the gut microbiome for better health. The innovations we've seen so far are just the beginning, and the next decade promises even more groundbreaking finds that will change the way we approach health and wellness.

The future of gut health is not just about treating symptoms but about optimizing and personalizing care, making it possible for people to thrive with a healthy, balanced gut microbiome. By staying informed and embracing these innovations, we can all look forward to a future where gut health plays an even more important role in achieving a longer, healthier life.

Glossary: Key Terms and Concepts

Understanding the terminology related to gut health is important for navigating the complex world of the microbiome, digestion, and general well-being. Here's a glossary of key terms and ideas to help you grasp the language of gut health and its many facets.

1. Microbiome

The collection of trillions of bacteria, viruses, fungi, and other microbes living in and on your body, especially in the gut. These microorganisms play a crucial part in digestion, immunity, and different bodily functions.

2. Gut Microbiota

The specific population of microorganisms living in the gut. This population includes a wide variety of bacteria, some beneficial and others possibly harmful. A healthy gut microbiota helps digestion and immune function.

3. Dysbiosis

An imbalance or disruption in the gut microbiota, often resulting from factors like poor diet, stress, drug use (especially antibiotics), or illness. Dysbiosis is linked to several health problems, including gastrointestinal disorders, autoimmune diseases, and even mental health issues.

4. Prebiotics

Non-digestible food components, usually fiber or complex carbohydrates, that promote the growth and activity of beneficial bacteria in the gut. Prebiotics are found in foods like garlic, onions, bananas, and whole grains.

5. Probiotics

Live microorganisms, mainly bacteria, that confer health benefits when consumed in adequate amounts. Probiotics can help restore the balance of good bacteria in the gut and are widely found in fermented foods like yogurt, kefir, sauerkraut, and kimchi.

6. Psychobiotics

A class of probiotics that may have a positive effect on mental health. Research suggests that certain probiotics can affect the gut-brain axis and help alleviate symptoms of anxiety, depression, and stress.

7. Gut-Skin Axis

The connection between the gut microbiome and the skin. An imbalance in the gut microbiota can add to skin conditions like acne, eczema, and psoriasis, while a healthy gut can promote clearer and healthier skin.

8. Gut-Brain Axis

The bidirectional communication system between the gut and the brain, combining neural, hormonal, and immune pathways. The gut microbiome can affect brain function, mood, cognition, and mental health, and vice versa.

9. Immune System

The body's defense system against dangerous pathogens, infections, and diseases. The gut microbiome plays a vital part in immune system regulation, as a big portion of the immune system is located in the gut.

10. Inflammation

A natural immune reaction to injury or infection, but when chronic, inflammation can lead to various diseases. Dysbiosis in the gut is often associated with chronic inflammation, which may lead to conditions like heart disease, diabetes, and autoimmune disorders.

11. Metabolism

The process by which the body turns food into energy. A healthy gut microbiome supports efficient digestion and absorption of nutrients, which in turn supports healthy metabolism and weight control.

12. Prebiotic Fiber

Types of fiber found in plant-based foods that are especially fermented by the beneficial bacteria in the gut. These fibers serve as food for probiotics, helping them thrive and keep a healthy gut environment.

13. Gut Permeability (Leaky Gut)

A disease where the lining of the intestines becomes damaged, leading to increased permeability. This allows harmful substances to leak into the bloodstream, triggering inflammation and adding to conditions like autoimmune diseases and digestive disorders.

14. Antibiotic Resistance

The power of bacteria to resist the effects of drugs that once killed them. Overuse or misuse of antibiotics can disrupt the gut microbiome and lead to the development of antibiotic-resistant bacteria, which pose a major health risk.

15. Gut Healing

The process of restoring balance to the gut microbiome, often after damage caused by illness, bad diet, stress, or antibiotic use. Healing the gut may involve dietary changes, prebiotics, probiotics, and other lifestyle tweaks.

16. Fecal Microbiota Transplant (FMT)

A medical procedure that includes transferring fecal matter from a healthy donor to a recipient's intestines. FMT has shown good results in treating conditions like Clostridium difficile infections and is being explored for other gut-related diseases.

17. Biofilm

A protective layer made by clusters of bacteria in the gut. Biofilms can keep dangerous bacteria from being eliminated by the immune system or antibiotics, leading to chronic infections and gut imbalances.

18. Microbial Diversity

The range of different microbes (bacteria, fungi, viruses, etc.) in the gut. A diverse microbiome is associated with better health outcomes, as it helps the gut and immune system work more effectively.

19. Gastrointestinal (GI) Tract

The set of organs responsible for digestion, including the stomach, small intestine, large intestine (colon), and rectum. The GI tract houses the majority of the body's microbiota, which plays a key part in digestion, nutrient absorption, and immune function.

20. Short-Chain Fatty Acids (SCFAs)

Fatty acids created by beneficial bacteria during the fermentation of fiber. SCFAs are important for gut health as they help reduce inflammation, strengthen the gut lining, and provide energy to cells in the gut.

21. Colonization Resistance

The ability of the gut's beneficial bacteria to keep harmful microbes from establishing themselves. A balanced gut microbiome stops pathogenic bacteria from taking over and causing infections.

22. Bile Acids

Compounds made by the liver to help digest fats. Bile acids are also involved in regulating the gut microbiome and can affect the composition of gut bacteria.

23. Gut Flora

Another term for the bacteria that live in the digestive system. It is often used interchangeably with gut microbiome, though it can refer to the bacterial component alone.

24. Antioxidants

Compounds found in certain foods that help fight oxidative stress and inflammation. Antioxidants like vitamin C, vitamin E, and polyphenols can help protect the gut and skin from damage caused by free radicals.

25. Prebiotic Foods

Foods that are rich in prebiotic fibers, such as garlic, onions, asparagus, bananas, and whole grains. These foods feed the beneficial bacteria in the gut and help keep a balanced microbiome.

26. Fermented Foods

Foods that have been through a process of fermentation, such as yogurt, kimchi, cabbage, and kefir. Fermented foods are natural sources of probiotics and can help support a healthy gut bacteria.

This glossary should help clarify some of the essential terms linked to gut health, probiotics, prebiotics, and the microbiome. Understanding these concepts is crucial for navigating the science behind gut health and making informed decisions about food and lifestyle to support your microbiome.